The African Holistic Motivational Healing Guide

Heal Our African Nation

The African Holistic Motivational Healing Guide

Heal Our African Nation

By Kevin Montez Forrest

The African Holistic Motivational Healing Guide

By Kevin Montez Forrest

Editor:Kevin Forrest
First Printing: August 2003

Manufactured in the United States of America
Black African Egyptian Studies\ Spirituality\ Self Help\ Personal Growth\ Higher Consciousness\ Health
ISBN 0-9743699-0-X
($ 9.95)

Published By
Kevin Forrest
761 North 80th Street
East St. Louis, IL. 62203

THE AFRICAN HOLISTIC MOTIVATIONAL HEALING GUIDE

Table of Contents

THE AFRICAN HOLISTIC MOTIVATIONAL HEALING GUIDE

Knowledge of Self

Heal Our African Nation!

Preface

I am an average person that started a quest for better health and awareness. I am not a Doctor or other Health specialist. I started my quest for Truth one day when I awoke and immediately had this strong desire not to go to work, so I followed my conscious mind and called work and took a day off. I did not know why I did this but now I needed something to do so I decided to try to catch up with my best friend, with whom I could never seem to catch. I arrived at his home and to my surprise, he was there. He took me to an African apparel shop where I received information on the Pyramids and the African's contributions to the world. And now, six years later, I have written this guide to share what has become the Truths in my life. Your health and well-being is in your hands. You don't need hundred's of educational degrees to determine what is good for your body. You must first learn that your mind soul and body are all under your control. You have every right to ingest all the mental, physical and spiritual knowledge that you can obtain from friends, family, books, tapes, lectures, video's etc… Then you must decide what of the knowledge is Truth in respect to you. And once this true knowledge has been obtained you must utilize as much of it in your every day life as you can.

This book gives Black people a method to get back to our Blackness and Black African way of life. I am writing this motivational guide in an attempt to raise the conscious level of the average man through her/his mental, physical and spiritual state of being. And to reestablish the weakened link between man and his spirit self (God Self). Also to put man back in tune and in harmony with his Spirit Self (God Self), which would put man back in tune with nature as the creator intended.

We must put the Feminine essence back into our World. Until this is done we will have a system that lacks one of its major components, like a car without an engine, like a computer without a processor, like living without spirituality and all the other gifts that she brings.

These health tips are from the Ancient ways of our Khametic Ancestors, basically speaking of our Egyptian fore Mothers and Fathers, who were vegetarians and the creators of the first Way of Life (Spiritual) System.

The Thought Process

When reading information or acquiring knowledge of any kind a person must first acquire the information then process this information. To process information a person must ask her or his self various questions about the data such as where did the information come from, what was the person's purpose when giving this information, and many other questions. After going through the process of analyzing the information one must conclude if the information is true or false or if they or indifferent about the data. This method will enable a person to formulate his or her own truths about the information which they have obtained, giving them a much better understanding of the information. Also you will be building a truth table in your mind that will aid you in obtaining more and higher Truths. One must never just accept information as true for if you do this you will be as a machine accepting what is given to you and never really knowing if it is true or not or really what the information is trying to convey to you. It is better to read five pages of a book in one hour and obtain one truth from the processing of this data, than to read fifty pages and have not obtained any truths from the information.

Heal Your Body Holistically

A person must first gather Health knowledge through picture's, articles, books, tapes, lectures, video's, friends, media and other forms of information. Now once you understand what good health is and how to maintain it. You can take the necessary steps: eat the right food and drink, get an exercise routine, fast, take enema's, think positive thoughts, pray. If you fail to follow your routine don't quit just try again no one is perfect. And for the fact that you have tried you are on your way to success and better health.
You are the best doctor for your body if you would just try to be, by learning and practicing good health. And paying attention to the signals that your body gives you, relating to good health or illness.
We must always realize if God gave us this body, do you think that he wanted us to abuse it. He wanted use to use it for the tasks that it was meant to perform.

I have noticed that in all the information I have gathered and reviewed that they keep stating that one must fast, purify, exercise, do enemas, think positive, pray and learn as much as possible about each. This will aid you in your quest for better health (mental, physical and spiritual). We will learn more about each of these later.

By purifying your body and mind you move towards a higher Physical, Mental and Spiritual state of being, giving you better health, state of mind and spiritual awareness.

We must use the things God gave us in nature to heal ourselves and keep use in a proper physical, mental, and spiritual state of being. Eat live foods and juices which have been touched by the sun and that have not loss their life giving essence. (The sun gives life force energy to the plants and we eat the plants and fruits, herbs and nuts!). You don't eat the animals that eat the plants this is second hand food (contains no life force energy in it). Try not to eat processed foods as this is second hand food. Get as much sun as possible to receive the life force energy direct from the sun light. And black people will not get cancer from the sun light. Black people bodies contain high levels of melanin which enables them to receive and process sun light into vitamin "D" and boost their immune systems. Also when the sunlight reacts to the melanin and water in your skin the sunlight's energies are separated and distributed throughout the body and aids organs and all bodily functions. The Sun's life force energy is infused into the water, air and soil. We must also understand that the body and all things are made of electromagnetic energy at different vibratory rates or frequencies. Since the body is electric in nature our first source of food is the Sun's electro magnetic energy and our second source of food is the air for which the Sun has infused its energy into the air molecules that we breathe to keep us alive. And third is the fresh unprocessed water which has the sun's energy stored up in it. Forth is the vegetation: fruits, vegetable, nuts, rice and other natural foods that have the Sun's life force energy stored in them.

You also need to take walks or stand on the earth or ground. The ground stores up the life force energy's within its self then re-emits it constantly throughout the day. And don't forget taking deep breaths as much as possible throughout your day because the sun embeds these life force energies into the air molecules . Then you breathe it in and extract this life force energy and it is carried throughout your body in your blood stream. You get the best quality of air during mid-day when the life-force energy from the sun is at its peak. Try to open windows as much as possible to let in fresh air. Also get more plants in your home, plants release oxygen, for you to breath. And don't forget prayer. Note you must fast and do enemas, because the air and food and water are polluted. Pollutants and parasites are the main two causes of bad health in our nation. Pollutants can cause parasites. Pollutants are in the food, air, hygiene, facial and skin care products etc...

Africans had the best health and knowledge system ever recorded in history. Wouldn't you like to follow the health practices of your Ancestors?

Forgive all those people whom have wronged you in your life. This is good mentally because you are not holding in any anger. And you are now thinking with your heart bringing out the love essence in you. Also you are thinking in a holistic manner for all of mankind. This will also cleanse your mental thought patterns, preventing you from thinking negative things that only cloud your mental progress.

Eating utensils should be made of stainless steal, glass, cast iron, clay. Don't use plastics and aluminum.
Plastic and aluminum utensils put pollutants such as formaldehyde in your body and large amounts of aluminum in your body causes malfunctions of the nervous system which includes the brain.

When eating always keep in mind how the body works from 4am-12noon the body detoxes (cleans) itself, from 12noon-7pm the body receives nutrients (food), and from 7pm-4am the body extracts the nutrients from the food.

Always remember that exercise enhances your organ's ability to do work, therefore rendering better overall body functions.

Having good physical health is easy. Just reduce the amount of toxins, poisons and non-natural substances entering the body and eat fresh whole foods and get as much sunshine and fresh air as you can.

Enema (Personal experience)

I was informed by multiple sources that I needed to perform an enema to insure good health. Immediately after performing my first hot water bottle enema, I felt a beautiful cleansing sensation run through my body from my head down to my toes. It felt so great I wanted to run down the street and scream it out to everyone in the neighborhood that they should do one. My skin looked so much better, I got a wonderful feeling in my head, much less fatigue in muscle and better breathing when exercising, I digested my foods so much easier. Note: please don't use hot water when performing an enema only warm water.

Fasting

Fasting is a great way to heal the body of illnesses, and dis-ease. Also it will cleanse and put the body at ease. There or several types of fast: Air fast (no food or drink), Water fast (fast on only spring and or mineral water, fruit juices), vegetable (fresh, uncooked), fruit and Nuts fast. When fasting one should always keep in mind that man is a three dimensional being physical, mental and spiritual.

Therefore, physically you should do your fast for the length of time that you have prescribed for your self and you should develop some sort of exercise program to go along with your fasting. Walking or running is good because it stimulate various nerve points in the foot that correspond to various organs in the body which promotes healing, release of tension, better circulation, etc. Also, Tai-Chi, Judo, Karate are other exercises that were created by the Black Egyptian Priest for maintaining good health. You should always try to get as much sun as possible because the sun is the key to all living things. One should, after fasting, try to start a vegetarian/fruitatarian type of every day diet because the only foods that man was meant to eat are the foods (raw, uncooked) that the sun touches and instills its life force energies into. One should also try to lower the amounts of salt, sugar and high calorie foods that we eat. Mentally you should read various literatures on fasting so that you will mentally understand the fasting and what to expect from it. Also talking to others will give you more mental understanding that will aid you in completing your fast. Spiritually you should meditate and pray that the creator will give you the energy and mental understanding to get you through your fast. You can fast as much as you like. One good time to fast is during seasonal changes as it will aid the body in adapting to the seasonal change. Also try to take warm baths to promote detoxification (cleansing) of the body and relaxation. You can use Epsom salt, lemon juice, lemon peels or apple-cider vinegar in your bath to aid in cleansing the body.

In the Ancient Black Egyptian society fasting was a common way of life, which helped to promote the quality and length of life. Try to restrain from sexual intercourse during your fast in order to keep your energies (physical/ mental/ spiritual) at there highest levels. When ill or injured you should fast. If you or a person that is under the care of a physician you can consult a physician (Naturopathic Doctor) before attempting to fast. When coming off of a fast one should not consume large amounts of food she/he should slowly raise there consumption back to a comfortable level. Note that while fasting you will become calmer and more accepting of your environment. During the fasting part of the diet the body gathers up its energy. Herbs and certain food were used to excite or stimulate the body's energies after fasting.

Monthly Fast

A good fasting program is to fast for three days straight per mouth. During this three day fast you can drink this Distilled Water or Apple Juice Mixture: Mix and drink while on fast, 1gallon water or apple juice, ½ teaspoon cayenne pepper, maple syrup (grade C) and one fresh squeezed lemon. You may at first want to fast one day per week then work up to the three day fast. While fasting, your body will get rid of poisons (toxins) that have been in your body for years, the longer you fast the more poisons you get out of your body.

People who have been on a vegetarian diet don't tend to feel bad when fasting because their body's or much cleaner inside and can adjust to the change much easier. It has been said that if you fast regularly you will get rid of bad ailments such as High blood pressure, Allergies, Acne, Arthritis, and a large number of other ailments.

You should mentally view your fasting in a positive light, always think and tell your self positive things while fasting, such as my body is being cleansed of waste products the more I fast. You should do enema's while fasting because your body releases more waste products during fasting and they or all sitting in your lower intestines and need to be flushed out of your body.

Drink fresh lemon juice while fasting, it will aid in the removal of mucus in your body. No milk products or meat while fasting. Try to drink at least 8 or 9 glasses of clean (if using tape water boil it first) water while on fast and after fast. You should slowly come off of your fast by slowly returning to your daily diet. But don't start back eating the bad foods that you ate before the fast (meat, milk products, candy, processed foods, soda, etc.) and this will help your body to stay clean in the long run. Find a good tea to drink while fasting. If after your fast you eat some of the foods that are not good for your body, you should take an enema and fast. Drink plenty of liquids, try to just eat fruits for a day, take a hot bath 15-30min and exercise. This will aid you in getting the toxins from the bad food out of your system.

Your blood receives its nutrients threw the intestines. If your intestines are full of toxins and poisons, your blood is full of toxins and poisons. And your blood receives oxygen threw the lungs and if the lungs are full of mucus from trying to get rid of the bad substances that you have eaten or breathed in, then you will not have the proper oxygen that is needed in the blood.

Fasting aids the body in balancing out its energies. The drinking of water while fasting helps the body to regain its balance. Remember the body is aprox. 90% water so drink plenty of water. Try to use distilled or spring water. You should prepare for and end your fast with a fruit, vegetables and liquid diet, one to two days before and after your fast. This will ease your body into and out of the fast and lower the amount of shock to the system. Physical exercise and deep breathing exercises while fasting will aid the body in cleansing and adjusting its energies to their correct levels. You can take herbs while fasting. It takes approximately three days of fasting to get all of the waste products out of your body.

Examples of Fast :

* May, 2001
I took a 3 day all liquid fast, around May, 2001 and exercised

* June, 2001
Fruit and nut fast 12 days, also exercise and meditation. It felt great.

* October 6, 2001
5 day fast: on the 6th I fasted and ate fruit that night, I ate fruit on the 7,8,9,10(ate dinner) and I have done four enema's and still doing my work out, and some meditation.

* October 27, 2001
Monthly 3 Day Fast. I COMPLETED a" 3 day Water Only" fast on distilled water and boiled water, cayenne powder, fresh lemon, and grade "A" molasses. I have made it through 27th , 28th, 29th day,- I have done meditation on the 1st, 2nd, 3rd day, also I exercised, sun-bathed, and took enema's each day. I started on the 26th at 9:00PM and ended on the 29th at 6:00PM.

Exercise

Exercise should be used to get your blood flow and circulation up in order to stimulate the functions of the organs and purify the body. Extreme exercise is not required for good heath. Examples of good exercises are, stretching all muscles, dancing, singing while standing, walking or jogging, Tai Chi, etc. Also you should exercise so that the skin can sweat out impurities from your body and cleanse it.

Diet (or dieting tips)

Avoid eating pork, shrimp, chicken, catfish, and lobster. These animals purpose on this Earth is to remove undesirable waste from the Earth. Therefore their bodyies are full of toxins and poisons and should not be eaten. Eat what is good for you; not what is good to you.
Herbal tea's don't mix sweeteners with your herbal tea's. It will decrease the effectiveness of the tea.

Stop practicing up and down dieting; eat a lot today; diet tomorrow. This only hurts the body and mind.
A lot of people keep their house cleaner than there bodies.

The most valuable things in life is good health. If you don't have good health how can you enjoy anything else?

Runny Nose / Sneezing

For runny nose (mucus secretion) eat a mix of lemons, oranges and grapefruits. Mucus is secreted when the body is trying to rid its self of waste or toxins. You need to get rid of mucus causing foods they stop your body from processing oxygen correctly. Such as pork, bread, pasta's etc. Here is a list of Herbs that can be taken to rid the body of mucus; Milk Thistle, Dandelion Root, White Pine, Wild Cherry, Colts Foot and Hyssop.

Waste Elimination

Always remember that if you eat three meals a day you should use the rest room (have a bowel movement) three times that day to remove waste products from your body. I now have one very large bowel movement in the morning and maybe another during the day. To aid your body in cleansing, you can drink one teaspoon of apple cider vinegar in water, every other day.

Bad Foods

Don't eat fried foods. They are constipating and hard for the body to digest. Also white sugar lacks nutrients, acts like a drug in your system and raises the sugar level in your body. Processed salt acts like a drug in your system, causes high blood pressure and causes the person to retain water in their body. Also processed salt has a damaging effect on the glands in the body. Bleached white flour is bad for you because it is constipating and has no fiber or nutrients in it. Various foods that contain preservatives and dyes are bad for your system such as candy bars, soda's, and a lot of the packaged foods in your grocery store. Don't eat canned foods, they may contain the metals (such as aluminum, and tin) that they are canned in. These metals are toxic and can interfere with your nervous systems functions. Processed foods are bad for you because the natural structure of the food has been changed due to the processing methods. Coffee and Cocoa contain caffeine which is bad for your system, especially your nervous system and body's Ph-balance.

Green Life Formula's

Everyone needs to start using a green life formula (Wheatgrass, Spirulina, Psyllium Husk, Barley etc…) they are very good for your system. These green formula's will detoxify (rid it of toxins) the body. Some people can't take a lot at first (may cause diarrhea) so you need to slowly get your intake up to an appreciable amount. Green plants and herbs balance and stimulate the electrical systems of the body.

Fresh green foods such as salads (lettuce, not cooked) provides the body with Chlorophyll which cleans and detoxifies the entire body. The chlorophyll in plants aids the plant in storing up the life force energy from the Sun. Now you receive this life force energy better when you eat fresh non-cooked green foods.

Green foods such as salads (green leaf) herbs (Spirulina, Parsley) etc. should be eaten all the time because they aid in keeping the electrical part of your body balanced and will correct it if it gets unbalanced. Also green foods should be eaten in the winter when the sunlight is less intense and most people don't get a lot of sun energy to feed their bodies. (Examples: Queen Afua's Heal Thyself Green Life Formula, Dr. Hagiwara's "Magnum Plus" or Garden of Life's "Perfect Food Super Green Formula")

Miracle Substances

Apple Cider Vinegar and Garlic are said to be Miracle Cures. A teaspoon of Apple cider vinegar or a pinch of fresh garlic each day will aid your body functions and cleanse your system. Note of caution: some people can not take a large amount of garlic; it lowers their metabolism. Also Onions or fresh lemons or fresh squeezed lemon juice and water are good for cleansing and bodily functions. Garlic will boost your Immune system, fights off bacteria and viruses, opens arteries, kills funguses in the body.

Processed Foods

Processed foods only exist because they generate money for big business. These same processed foods will destroy the body over an extended period of time (will cause disease and or shorten your life span). Also don't eat fried foods. The frying of the food is a type of processing that produces substances not normally meant to be eaten. The bad dietary practices that we have are like chemical warfare on our bodies.

Diet

Black people have a different dietary requirement than White people such as the fact that a large number of Black people can not digest milk. They have lactose deficiency; their body stopped producing the substance which is requireded to digest milk. Pasteurized milk lacks the enzymes, vitamins, and minerals needed for good health. A lot of peoples in other lands do not consume dairy foods. In nature, once an animal is out of the infant stage they no longer drink milk. Blacks have an extremely small amount of the enzyme required to digest meats, therefore meats stay in our systems longer (up to 10 days or more) and spoils. But Whites have a larger amount of this enzyme. Black people's blood content is not the same as Whites. Our digestive systems are the same as they were when we lived in Africa. So we should eat an African vegetarian type of diet. White's digestive systems or different from Blacks, so the two races digest there foods differently and require different foods.

When the body has too many toxins, it uses urination, defecation, sinuses (mucus) and skin (bumps and discolorations) to rid itself of these toxins. Bad food and chemicals act like drugs in your body, uppers and downers. We must search for the proper diet, good foods that will give you balance and peace mentally physically and spiritually. Your taste for foods will change if you keep eating different foods from that which you ate before.

Water

Water helps the human body to absorb and distribute the proper minerals and life force energy. So drink plenty of clean fresh water and this will aid your body in keeping proper mineral and energy balance at all times.

Climate

We were meant to live in a climate that has all that is needed to support the human life form such as Africa and other surrounding area's which have a similar climate. These climates are high in vegetation which brings forth a good quality of air, fruit and vegetables to eat and a warm climate so that you are not forced to live inside and can get the life giving essence from the Sun-Light into your body. It has been proven by scientist that the human body functions best at temperatures between 70-98 degree's Fahrenheit and that various parts of the body starts to shut down as the temperature decreases below 70 degree's.

Oxygen

Hydrogen Peroxide (H(2),0(2) molecule), pure oxygen(from a tank), and liquid Oxygen will all increase the bodies oxygen level and kill off bad bacteria in the body, also helps mental abilities. Also you can use Hydrogen Peroxide to clean your fruits before you eat them.

Most Advanced Genetic Structure

If all people except a small group from one race were to perish from the Earth then the only group that could repopulate the earth with all the different races is the black race. This is due to the scientific fact that they are the only race that caries all the genetic information for every race of people, which would be required to regenerate all the races. This genetic information also is what makes black peoples physical, mental and spiritual essence the oldest and most advanced on this planet.

Mental Health

Always remember that a lot of illnesses are the result of negative thinking such as worrying, stress, and thinking negatively when things don't go your way, and getting upset. A poor person worries about gaining things and a rich person worries about loosing things. You should always try to keep your mental state balanced and calm. When you are in this state, your mind and body will function at its best. You should try to hold this calm state even when happy, stressed, sad or upset so that your body and mind functions will not decrease. If they do, this is when disease will enter your body. Stress will impair the function of various glands and cause unregulated hormone releases resulting in sluggish felling (slowed metabolism), sleeplessness and emotional instability. Research has proved that the major cause of Heart-attacks is negative thoughts (thinking) such as feeling unhappy and feeling that your life has little or no purpose, "what you think, you shall become". The mind emits electromagnetic vibrations that we call thoughts. These thought vibrations evolve into more thoughts or physical actions. So in order to have good thoughts and actions we must cleanse our minds initial thoughts which will bring forth more good thoughts and good actions. Be sure that each time you start a new thought vibration that it is a positive thought. I will not perform mental and spiritual genocide upon myself or my people. I will cleans my thoughts.

You say that the Creator (God) exist and is within you and controls all yet you fear man and all the ills of the world that he has created. These ills result in stressing you out and lowering you physical, mental and spiritual health. Don't fear either man nor any of his ways; just meditate (pray) for mankind, and do the best you can in life.

Doing good things for others will develop your love for mankind, giving you a better disposition and state of being.

A person can find mental peace in knowing the Truths about the Past, Present and Future. A wise person has retrospect and is always searching for new Truths and is willing to give up old Truths if proven to be wrong. An unwise person assumes that they know all, they never review old Truths to see if they should be replaced with new Truths and is closed minded to any new truths. Or they just accept anything as a Truth.

Mind

There are two types of mental thought that each man possesses. One is Negative thought the other is Positive or righteous thought. Both forms of thought are given to us by God and are necessary in life. The negative side is the side that people who try to upset or hurt you use. The positive side is what makes a person relaxed or focused and act out of love for self and mankind. We must all work to use our positive or righteous thought to get us through every task, day and event in our lives and only then will we have constant peace of mind in our lives.

A good approach to proper thoughts and actions is to first be sure that you are outwardly living your life and not hiding from the ills of the world. Some people rarely leave their homes because they are afraid of the negative things in society. You were not given life to hide from living it. God gave each man and woman a purpose in life and we must get out there and live our lives so that we can find our purpose for living. Next we must use our best judgment when assessing various things in life and don't let jealousy, hatred, ego or other thing impair our good judgment. Third: we must search for the truths in all situations in life and act upon and build on this set of Truths each day of your life. Finally, when acting upon this set of truths in life, we must act out of love for self and all of humanity. Which can be termed as acting out of universal love for all and everything. Now in accordance to Gods law when you act out of love you receive love back. If this process is followed the person will raise her/his mental physical and spiritual state of being to their highest levels.

If possible, stop to help a stranger or a friend; you will get a good feeling from the heart after doing good deeds for others and the creator will smile down on you. These deeds are very necessary when trying to establish a proper spiritual mind set.

Negative things in our live are generated from the fears that we have "cause and effect". Fear is a negative outward act that brings negative things into your life, so don't fear just make good decisions. We must also realize that some things that we perceive to be negative are not. Example: I was wrongfully fired from my job even though I performed very well on the Job. I could have taken this off time negatively but I chose to be calm and I was able to write this book, turning a so called negative into a positive.

Calm State of Mind

Your temperament dictates your actions. So always keep a calm attitude towards life and you will always bring forth proper actions in all situations. Always remember that the best decision making is done with a calm mind. In an overly excited (happy) or sad (upset) state of mind we tend to make bad choices and our mental processing is not at its best. Also stress in the body leads to a failure or impairment of bodily functions. You can use Honeysuckle Oil for better thinking (brain functions) and memory. You become what you think: meaning that if you constantly feed your mind bad thoughts your physical actions will become bad in nature. If you constantly feed your mind righteous thoughts you will display righteous actions. Remember that the mind exist at a higher state than does the physical body and it has control over the body's functions so if you think bad or stressful thoughts your body's functions will be affected bringing about bad health and other ailments.

The mind and other organs in the body are negatively affected when a person feeds their body bad foods (foods that contain various toxins). The bodies organs are negatively affected in the same way as a drunken person stumbles and can't think straight due to the fact that the liquor has gone to their brain and is confusing the brains processing mechanisms. This liquor (toxic substance), has also had a bad affect on all the other organs in the body lessening their ability to do work. Therefore, remember bad foods are distributed throughout all organs in the body and cause ill effects on all the bodies organs.

Mentality

Black's people are suffering from racism in ways that have negative affects on their ability to make good, self derived decision. We believe all the lies that are ingested mentally by us through the media (TV, newspaper, commercials, radio, magazines), books, pictures, politicians, and preachers. We accept this data without trying to find out the source and objective of the person putting out the information. Then we accept this information as truths and now we base our life on all these non-truths, which throws off our whole physical, mental and spiritual purpose in life. We need to stop watching T.V. garbage and preoccupy our minds with positive thoughts. When I stopped watching T. V. and listening to the radio I notice that I felt more peaceful. I thought about and found the answer to a lot of my problems in life.

Maturing Mind

We must always remember that during puberty a child's glands start to produce more hormones and these hormones have a physical and mental (more sensitive) affect on the child. Natural eating is a must during this time because the child is developing physically, mentally and spiritually. Also, puberty is a time when by nature a child has now developed into an adult and by nature is ready to start the reproductive stage of life. But, we as parents have not taught the young adult how to handle these new instinctive sexual urges which have been brought on by these hormone changes. So the young adult blindly goes forth trying to figure out why he/she is so attracted to the opposite sex and what to do about it. We must teach the children about this change of mental state.

Black Mental Slavery

A smart slave (Black Doctor's, Preachers, the Average Black person, Politician's, Lawyers, etc.) can create me (the system) a whole society and run it for me, but not even know that he is part of the system. Now when we as Black's stop following the programmed way of thought and start thinking, creating and following our own thoughts then we stop being well paid or unpaid slaves and free our selves from the pains and wrongs of this society and start to create a new way of thought based on our Black culture, religion, and knowledge of all things. This should be first most in the black woman/man's mind, giving truth to the term "Know Thyself". Also remember to not be a person who always talks of doing good things but never puts these thoughts into action.

Melanin Increases with Age

The amounts of melanin in the brain increase with age. This is related to the terms the older the wiser, respect your elders. Therefore the older you get the more you become knowledgeable of your God self (Spirit Self, Third Eye).

Spiritual Heath

Practice meditation daily to clear the mind and pray to the creator to aid you in your positive thinking and way of life. Don't forget the spiritual side of life. Pray and read spiritual and spiritual healing books. Always pray while practicing better health measures. Ask God to return you to your Natural African mental state of mind. Every aspect of your life can be uplifted through meditative prayer. Be devoted to your spiritual essence, meditate on a regular basis, not just when things are going bad. To be balanced you must be physically mentally and spiritually balanced and if one of these or out of balance, then the other two will suffer. The physical body renews its self approximately every six to eight years. The speed at which the body renews is directly related to the vibratory rate of the individual or his conscious state of being. A person who has a higher conscious state of being (higher vibratory rate) will rejuvenate his/her body at a faster rate than that of lower conscious individuals. Use Camphor oil for better spiritual health. Also drink teas containing dandelion root or leafs.

Meditation

We should meditate (pray) several times a day (morning, noon, night), if possible. This is a self brain training or tuning technique where you train your mind to focus on the Spiritual thoughts of life, there by tuning your self to the God essence within you. The more you meditate the more you become in tune with the Oneness "God", "Creator" or God self. You are tuning your body and mind to transmit and receive in the spiritual realm of life, where all truths will be revealed to you.

Churches

Churches need to get back to their proper function which is Physical, Mental and Spiritual guidance. Not play acting, ego tripping, modeling of clothing, woman/man chasing and making money. The church needs to stop being the Social club or bar (without the liquor).

Colon

From news on TV, the 2nd leading cause of cancer is colon cancer (cancer of the anus) . We need to do enemas to prevent this. When you do a colon cleansing or hot water bottle enema you eliminate a large amount of toxins, worms and poisons from your body which could later in life cause serious health problem. Also this cleansing will increase your circulation.
There exist pathways from the colon to every organ in your body therefore you should clean the colon and have a healthy diet so that toxins and poisons will not find their way through these pathway to you organs and cause them to malfunction and become diseased.

This type of cleansing will reduce the chances of the occurrence of tumors and other ailments of the reproductive organs, breast etc.... The consumption of milk products have been said to cause ailments in the reproductive organs such as tumors. Milk is not good for your bones and may causes Osteoporosis (bone and joint disease). You can take the herb "Horsetail' to strengthen your bones hair ands nails. If you have problems relating to your reproductive organs eat Okra, it is good for these organs. Also there exist points in your feet that correspond to every organ in your body. If you have pains in your feet this could be a sign that some organ in your body is ailing and needs to be put back at ease (cured of an ill condition).

Breast Feeding of Infants

A mother should breast feed her infant because the milk has been created by her body with the proper balance of nutrients for the baby's growth and well being. Also a mother should eat the proper foods as mentioned in the above dieting section. This will reduce the baby's chances of disease, allergies and other ill effects. We must note that cow's milk was meant for cows to consume, not for humans. Mothers milk is meant for humans. And that processed milk and other processed foods are also bad for an infant or breast feeding mother. A mothers body automatically cleans and purifies itself when pregnant so the mothers milk and body are clean and free of toxic substances.

Breathing Exercises

Perform deep breathing exercises at least once in the morning and once at night, this will aid in relaxing, balancing and uplifting your body and mind. You should breath air in through your nostrils down into your stomach and out of your mouth. The sun puts its life force energy into the air, so you should do deep breathing exercises so that you get more of this life force energy into your bodies. Your body will use this energy for physical, mental and spiritual endeavors such as healing the body, producing positive thought patterns and linking you to your Spirit-Self. Also this will put more oxygen into your body which aids your body in the distribution of nutrients. This process will aid all organs ability to do work. Also, it will increase the minds ability to process data (think). Please remember that air-conditioned air is processed air and is not good for the body. Example: You should sit near a window or outside under the Sun and first relax the mind. Then you should take a deep breath through the nostrils, for about 4 seconds. Then hold this same breath for about two seconds allowing the life force energy to be removes from the air and circulated into your body. Now exhale all of this air for about four seconds. Now give yourself a two second pause and then repeat this process. This will give you a good rhythmic breathing pattern. You can increase the time as you get better at deep breathing. While performing this exercise you must repeatedly tell your mind and body that you are pulling in life force energy and sending this life force energy throughout the entire body. You can also try to picture in your mind, the life force energy entering your nose and then being carried throughout the entire body. When I first started practicing the above breathing exercise my stomach did not fell well and it was tossing and turning, but when I finished the breathing exercise I felt energized and my stomach troubles had gone away. Ancient masters say that to increase brain power you should deep breath through one nostril while holding the other closed. Then deep breath threw the second nostril while holding the first nostril closed. Now repeat this pattern of breathing several times.

Aging

It is well know in the health society that the human body should not grow old due to the fact that the body can repair any damage that is done to it. Therefore a person of 75 years of age should feel and be able to do the things that a person of 20 can do. What you do to your body is what causes this so called aging affect not time. Just as your body heals from a minor cut, burn, bruise, broken bone, head or stomach ache, your body can heal itself from any other bodily ailment or disease, by way of proper health care and mental state of mind and meditative prayer. You are what you eat and think and spiritually manifest yourself to be.

Clothing

The body requires proper flow of fluids throughout the body such as blood, and spinal fluid etc... Don't wear tight clothing because tight clothing will restrict the flow of fluids throughout the body and may cause various ailments. This is the same way that fatty foods clog your arteries and restrict the flow of blood to the heart.

Love Making

Cleans yourself before love making. Clean the body not only on the out side but within (fasting, enema, etc.) and always think positive loving thoughts while love making. The child that you produce is a product of what the mother and father are physically mentally and spiritually. A proper mental and spiritual state will bring forth a higher evolved soul into your new born child. Always use meditative prayer to bring the proper mate to you. Cleanliness is next to Godliness so bring a God-Child into this world.

Make-ups / Cosmetics

Most make-ups (and nails polishes etc.) contain toxins such as pork products and other harmful chemicals that or being absorbed into your body by the skin. A good diet will help you to look better without all the bodily damage that cosmetics promote.

Colognes

People should use the various pure oils, such as Honeysuckle Oil, as perfumes and colognes to scent the body because a lot of the perfumes and colognes contain substances that are absorbed through your skin and are bad for your health.

Bathing

You can use a few drops of Lavender, Lemon, Pine and or Eucalyptus essential oils in your bath. These oils are good for the skin and body. Try to get essential oils because they are a more pure form of oil. One other good point to mention is that baptism was performed to reintroduce more life force energy into the body giving the person more natural healing ability and vigor. Life force energy was stored up in the water by way of the sun or from the earth's energy. Earth energy is the Sun's energy that has been stored up in the Earth. This energy radiates from the Earth all day but most of this energy is forced into the Earth during daylight hours by the Sun and is reemitted at night. (this is why some summer nights or so hot.)

Also Mineral Salts, Lemon juice or peals and Apple cider vinegar can be used to clean the skin and open pores.

Deodorant

Don't use deodorants that contain Aluminum Chlorohydrate, Aluminum derivatives or other harmful chemicals, Aluminum cause the bodies electrical (nervous) systems to malfunction. A good deodorant to use is the Thia Crystal Deodorant Stone which works well and last a long time. Its only ingredient is Mineral Salts.

Microwave Ovens (radiation)

Microwave ovens are not good to cook in. The waves from the microwave-oven will kill the vitamins and minerals contained in the food leaving you with a dead food which contains no vitamins or minerals. Also microwave ovens put small amounts of harmful radiation in your food and the surrounding atmosphere. Today radiation is being used on meats in the processing plant to kill the bad things in the meat such as viruses and bateria, but after this process the meat contains radiation which is bad for your body.

Medical Industry

The medical industry has problems. Doctors were giving patients experimental drugs with out the patient's permission. A heart patient had to get a pacemaker after he was given experimental drugs. And they gave these drugs to a pregnant woman. The Doctor and Staff falsified Patients records buy giving their own urine and blood samples in place of the patients, so that they could get paid aprox.16,000, 20,000 up to 200,000 from the research companies. These experimental drugs are reviewed by a panel that the drug manufacturer chooses, so that their drug will be approved for public use and they get millions of dollars.

** Melanin **

Melanin - the substance or chemical found in the skin of Black people that gives them there dark complexion. It is also found in various organs of the body, brain, glands and in the nervous system.
"Kem" is the African name for Melanin which mean infused with spirit. Melanin is what gives you strength physically, mentally, and spiritually as shown below. Black people have the most advanced DNA chain of all races on this earth which leads them to be the most advanced of the human species. In the formation of the human body Melanin tells the bodies DNA how to construct the human body.

Energy Storage

Melanin is found in the plants, animals, water and soil; this leads me to believe that it is a necessary and major component in life. The largest amounts of Melanin are found in the skin which is an organ in the human body. Black people have a highly Melanated Nervous system, starting at the Pineal Gland then to the Brain down through the spine and out to each and every nerve ending in your body. The Black color of Melanin allows it to store up energy (physical, mental and spiritual energies). Examples of the kinds of energy stored (or absorbed into) in melanin is the Sun's life force energy, sound energy (Music), mental energy, sunlight energy, Spiritual energy, Earth's magnetic energy or all stored up in your Melanin like a battery stores up electricity. This ability to store energy allows a Black person to receive energy from various sources and then use this energy for the various physical, mental and spiritual functions of the Body. We must protect our Melanin by proper diet, exercise, proper thinking and meditative prayer, so that our body can function at it's best. Always get lots of sun energy in the summer (sun tan) to increase the amounts of melanin in your body. Melanin increases ones ability to fight off disease. It increases the Immune System functions.

Melanin even has the ability to reproduce itself. A person should ingest the proper nutrients through the skin or mouth which contains the substance needed to create more melanin. One major nutrient needed is the mineral copper, so wear your copper jewelry in the winter when less sunlight energy is available. Tyrosine is an Amino Acid used by the body in the production of Melanin. This substance can be found in "Brewers Yeast" and other dietary supplements. Please take these supplements to keep your melanin levels high and especially during the winter months.

Melanin is a chemical that regulates all bodily functions and sustains life. The Brain communicates to the whole body by way of the Melamine contained in your skin, nerve's and cells of your body. Melanin acts like a copper wire, phone line and or power cord carrying data and energy throughout the body.

This country spends large amounts of money each year for the study of Melanin. You can do a search on the Internet and you will find many articles etc... on Melanin research. (search for "Journal of Pigment Cell Research", "Journal of Pineal Research ", " Journal of Nero-Transmition").

Black people have highly sophisticated and complex bodies. This is shown in our high level of mental and physical functions, well structured physical bodies, and spiritual nature. We have yet to move back to the highest level of society due mainly to our lack of knowledge of self, and our history, (African Egyptian ancestors).

Melanin in the scientific world is known as a super chemical due to its properties, such as its ability to be a super conductor of energy. The Egyptian translation of the word chemistry means the study of melanin.

Hospitals have machines and methods based on the white mans melanin level (the lowest) not the black mans (highest). Prosaic is a drug that stops the melanin in your body from working or carrying out its function. Whites people have a calcified pineal gland and this is why they don't produce as much melanin as Black people.

The Mesoderm of the brain is where the black dot or Third-Eye is located above the pineal gland, it is larger in black people, and this part of your brain connects you spiritually to the whole universe.

Melanin Absorption Ability / Drug Use

Melanin will chemically react to (or mix with) various drugs such as Marijuana, Alcohol, Cocaine, Cigarettes etc... This reaction causes the Black user of these products to have a decrease in the various body functions (physically mentally, and spiritually) including the brain and causes him to be highly addictive because his body now thinks that the drug he is using is melanin (a natural component of the body). These drugs mix (bond to) with your melanin and causes the drug to stay in your system longer. Also he will stay dependent on a drug for a longer time. Some of the legal drugs may have this same affect on black people. Some electrical frequencies can be harmful to melanated people, and this energy is being sent through your body from the various electrical components around you. Melanin is produced by your Pineal Gland (spiritual gland). Ancient one's called the pineal gland the cradle of God. The consumption of green plants keeps the Pineal Gland functioning at its highest level. The mixing of the Drug Cocaine with your body's melanin will eventually lead to a poisoning of the body and death. Don't use food as a drug; over eating is harmful to your health. Remember that a lot of the drugs that we ingest are substances that have been altered from their natural state. Our body's reactions to these unnatural substances are always some kind of ill effect. This is why we have so many side effects from taking the various drugs including doctor prescribed commercial drugs (aspirin, allergy medications, etc…).

The White man's body can not store up large amounts of energy like the Black mans Melanated body can and this lack of energy storage due to lack of melanin causes his body to function at a lower level than that of the Black Man's and therefore subjects him to more bodily disorders (physically, mentally and spiritually). Remember that a lot of White people or Blacks saying they or White, note how some so called Whites can tan(Black) but others can not(white). Historical, artifacts and human remains all show that the Black man and woman were on this planet before the white man so therefore all humanity should be classified as African people. Which leads use to the fact that their is only one race of people on this planet and all of the separating factors such as race, religion, class, wealth, country are only man-made and not based on facts or truths. Melanin can act like a conductor and will conduct electrical current but it also can act as an insulator and not allow current to pass through it. Melanin will also store up various minerals in the body, to use later in keeping the body-functioning. It is also involved in giving Black people the rhythmic abilities in dance and song. Melanin aids in the fast movement of the eye and all other muscles in your body, one reason for this is that the melanin passes the signal from brain to the muscle, at a faster rate through the black man/woman nervous system. Your entire body operates off electric signals from the brain. The Melanin in your body is the electric wire or conductor that sends and receives messages from the brain and environment. (The pineal gland uses copper to create melanin).

Lack of melanin in a pregnant woman may cause the woman to lose the child or the child may be born with a birth defect. This is why Blacks have a higher success rate when it comes to child births.

Melanin can cause altered states of consciousness such as telepathic communication, excited states such as that shown in black churches (shouting etc.), the trance-like state when dancing, raising of your Kundalini, or Third Eye. Melanin can act on it's own like a computer and control some bodily functions without referring back to the Brain for instructions.

Melanin is the reason why the Black Egyptian people were the most highly advanced society ever know to man, developing the science's, music, religion (truth seeking), mathematics, judicial systems (righteousness), Astrology (Astronomy), Medicines (herbs), Medicare (Healing). Melanin is responsible for keeping Black peoples mental state calm and relax, and not letting them move into a hostile or erratic state of mind. Nature (God) has given Black people a true gift when God gave us melanin. Melanin's affects on the brain causes Black people to think different than non Black races of people.. This lead you to the fact that Black's have different social and society structures. In nature if a certain things lacks color but another has color which would you say is the most advanced? When looking at different groups of Blacks around the world you will see that they all act alike (have the same mannerisms) this is due to the melanin in their brains which influences their thinking. Each person's melanin is receiving and responding to the same frequencies in the universe.

Melanin & Sports

Athletes are probably our best thinkers. But the system shows them in the public eye only as athletes, yet if you have superior message processing to the muscles you also have superior brain processing, both due to having a highly melanated nervous system(brain) and body. Example Jackie Joyner was an extremely good student in school (all A's) but the Media never talks of her in this manner. Another male Olympic Track Star is a physicist but this is never told to the public. The Media suppresses this information.

Melanin Types

The Melanin producing groups of people (type A produces the largest amounts of melanin).

Type A - Africans: Nubians, Nigerian, American Blacks, American Indians, Ethiopian, etc…
Type B - Indians, Puerto-Recan, Mexicans, Arabian etc….
Type C - Japanese, Chinese, Greeks, Italians etc….
Type D - Russians, Romans, Germans etc….

As you move up the types scale your melanin count goes up and your melanin related abilities go up!

When your body gets a cut on the skin melanin rushes to the cut and surrounds the damaged area, then the melanin induces it's frequency into the damaged area aiding in the repair of the cut. This is why Black people scar's are always dark in color. So increase your Melanin with more sun exposure and cure your self of all ill effects. Also melanin gives the skin an elastic nature so that it can stretch but not break.

Nature

If we let nature take its own course, we will note that the Black Female is the most Feminine woman (physically and mentally) on this planet. And the Black Male is the most masculine on this planet. Therefor all men shall be attracted to the Black woman and all Females to the Black male. And the Blacks highly melanated body will dominate over all others in most cases, giving the reason why the worlds population is predominately people of color. And a very small proportion of the population is white people.

Test on young children show that black kids or at a higher level due to the amounts of melanin in their brains. Now if you put all kids in the same class with no prejudice agenda (let nature take its own course) then the Black child will be seen as the smartest and the leader and also due to his fast physical development will be physically dominant. These test or kept hidden from the public.

The Pineal Gland

The Pineal Gland, the gland that produces the hormone called Melanin, is said to be the seventh sense that aids Black people in experiencing higher energy states (Raising of the Kundalinni or God self, telepathy, etc…). The Black Egyptian's utilized this state of being in every aspect of their lives. The production of Melanin increases with age in Blacks people, this increase is directly related to the fact that our elder or more spiritual and wiser, if their mental is in the correct state. More melanin in the brain in older Blacks gives them the ability to "See", (Use Third-Eye, Raise Kundalinni, To make more spiritually conscious). Note: see later section for more information.

History

African Health Practices were well established approximately 55,000 to 100,000 years ago and today's Western Medical Practice's were derived from this system but lost a lot of its effectiveness through commercialization and greed. Science has proved that these people were free of tooth decay and disease.
A Black Egyptian named Imhotep created the oldest Medical Science books on record. This medical system did not use machines as we do today in western medicine. The Imhotep Medical schools were called "Escalapian Temples". The Egyptian medical practice was based on disease prevention before the body has reached a disease state (unlike Western Medicine), by the use of good daily body, mind and spiritual up keep of the body. And they used methods for detecting dis-ease before a disease state was reached in the body. Over 17 volumes of medical science books were written by Imhotep, which are now in German educational facilities and have been given a new name, Ebers Papyrus. Ebers is the name of the European that stole and claimed Imhotep's works for his own.

African social structures had hospitals and were practicing all kinds of surgeries more than 3,000 years ago. The African Healing practices of the past were understood by all of it's people. Unlike the modern Western Medical system which the average man can not understand. A person can't even pronounce the names of the drugs they are taking let alone understand the effects the drug has on your body. European medicine treats mind, body and spirit separately where as African holistic health practices treat them as one (self). The three are all inter-connected parts of the body. The Egyptian mystery system medical students were educated for approximately 15 years in subject matter relating to all known aspects of physical, mental and spiritual state of being. Many civilizations (majority of the world) that had relations with Africa learned the holistic sciences of Africa and used them in their health practices. To day the African Sciences are very prevalent in the Asian sections of the world. The Ancient African's used color, natural foods, the body, oils, metals, incense, crystals, music, herbs, sun (life force energy), water, celestial bodies etc. in their holistic sciences. African Science is the oldest and highest level of science that you can find upon this planet and is the mother of all other sciences.

The African Priest took an oath not to teach any European's of the higher teachings of the Mystery System above the 3rd degree (science, Astrology, religion, math etc…), because the African's viewed the Europeans as an unstable group of people that would misuse this knowledge (today's so called modern world).

During the time of the slave trade European doctors use slaves to test their drugs and poisonous antidotes on, resulting in the death of many black people. And in modern times we still see this practice when recalling the Tuskegee Syphilis experiments that were performed on blacks.

Ancient Africans, due to their diets, lived well over 300 years of age. But the European lived only to approximately 40 years of age. Without the medicinal herbs and medical knowledge of Africa, the European race would have been over come by diseases in their societies.

Sunlight

When sun light (Electromagnetic energy) hits the body many frequencies of light (Electromagnetic Spectrum) are passed to the physical body through your melanated skin. Your conscious spiritual level and amount of melanin in the body determines how much of this life force energy (Sun light) your mind and body can interact with, store-up and use. This sunlight is transmitted into living matter and things and creates some of the vitamins and minerals needed for your body to function. This sunlight is infused into the air, so that it can be breathed into the body. Due to pollution some of our bodies can not perform this process as well as we did in Ancient times when air water and food were pure (in its proper state) and when our minds were less polluted with un-truths. The taking in of sun energy by the body can reverse the ill effects of drugs, bad diet, or poor thought processing. Also this energy can aid in the cleansing of the body and digestion of foods. Example: I was sun bathing in my car letting the sun rays penetrate my body from the waist up and each time after sun bathing I noticed that I would have a good bowel movement. After sunbathing on a regular basis I noticed that my body would sense when the sun was shining (high energy state) or when it was not (low energy state) even though I was inside a dark house. The taking in of Sun light is a physical, mental and spiritual healing agent for the black man/woman to cure themselves of disease or illnesses and maintain good health. Example: One day my knee was hurting very bad. I went out and sun bathed. After about five minutes I noticed that my knee had stopped hurting.

The Human Energy Cycle

The sun energy is received by man's body (and processed by way of the skin's melanin) and is then past down though the feet into the iron ore of the Earth' then back up from the Earth through the feet and body and back to the Sun, this is known as the "Human Energy Cycle". This cycle keeps the body constantly energized and grounded to the Earth and brings forth higher mental physical and spiritual abilities. Man should walk on the Earth as much as possible and wear no shoes or shoes with animal skin soles. Rubber soled shoes may break the energy cycle, because rubber is an insulator that the energy may not flow easily through.

Skin Cancer / Skin

I was told by a black doctor that there has only been one incident of skin cancer among black people and that was in a black albino person. Black Albino - a black person who has little or no melanin in his or her skin and body, giving them an extremely white complexion and light colored hair.

Oils

For cooking use "Virgin Olive Oils" (try not to over heat the oils) if it is going to be highly heated use peanut oil it can handle the higher heat (it will not change to another substance when heated) and will not break down. Don't eat Canola or other types of processed oils. Shea Butter is a good natural moisturizer to use on the skin or you can use Virgin Olive Oil.

Acupressure, Massage and Hands-on-Healing

Acupuncture, Massage, Acupressure and Hands-on-Healing were created and perfected by the Black Egyptian health systems. In the hands-on treatments the Black Egyptian Shaman or priest would, by use of hands and trained mental spiritual teachings would sense the person natural body frequency and then find where the body did not carry the right frequency and re-introduce the normal body frequency back into the body to cure the patient of their illness. The healer used the electromagnetic force contained in the Life Force Energy that She/He received from the Sun and the Air and transferred this energy from his body to the patient's body, and this input of energy is what heals. This electromagnetic force can be stored up in various substances or materials; the melanin in the skin and the water in the human body. Also the patient can be healed by treating the illness with herbs.

Various parts of the body are interrelated. If you put pressure on one part of the body and it hurts (finger, toe, heal of foot) then the organ that is related to that part of the body is ill (not at ease, or veered away from its normal energy state). This technique is part of the study of reflexology.

If possible, get a massage while fasting, either professional, from a loved-one or friend. A massage can relieve tension, pain, increase mental capabilities, invigorate you, calm nerves, increase circulation and flush toxins from your body. Massage also keeps the electrical nervous system of your body functioning properly allowing energy to flow through all parts of the body, bringing forth maximum brain and body activity and functions. Remember your body is electric. Massage your spouse or significant other each night.

Varicose Veins

Veins in the body can be harmed by meats and hydrogenated fats, salts and white sugar in your diet.

Cold, Flu's, Head Ache

Cold, Flu's, and Head Ache's are the body's way of letting you know that one or more of it's systems are not functioning properly due to toxins and pollutants in the system. When one of these warning symptoms occurs, fast, exercise, and cleanse your body.

Eyes

Your eyes require nourishment from the color spectrum in the rays of sunlight. So don't wear shades as they prevent the eye's from getting the needed nourishment.

Glands

The electromagnetic energy that you receive from sun light will stimulate and nourish the pituitary pineal and other glands of the body.

Sugar, Salt, Alcohol, Cigarettes

Sugar, salt, alcohol, and cigarettes are all addictive substances that should not be ingested into the body. A person should use Turbinado Sugar (natural raw cane sugar) in the place of processed white sugar and Celtic Sea Salt or Sea Salt in the place of processed salt. Honey or Sorghum can be used as a second choice in place of white processed sugar. Buckwheat and some dark honeys have a high antioxidant content which can aid the body in ridding its self of toxins. Don't use sugar substitutes some of them have disease causing chemicals in them and can be very harmful to the body!

White processed sugar will strip the body of vitamins and cause the body to try to get these loss nutrients from various organs. And the organs or weakened by this process, leading to poor digestion, and bodily functions. The consumption of sugar can have negative effects on the brain such as fatigue, Forgetfulness etc... It slows the immune system functions in the body. White sugar is found in so many of the food products found at the grocery store but you must reduce your consumption of white sugar by a lot or eliminate the use of white sugar if you want good health and long life. Sugar can cause kidney damage, contributes to cancers of the breast and organs, weakens eye sight, can cause heart disease, cause hemorrhoids, cause food allergies, weaken DNA and protein structure's in the body, and these or a few of sugars side effects.

Organs

The liver is used in the elimination of toxins from the body, for this reason animal livers is full of toxins and should not be eaten. And no animal organs should be eaten anyway. Also intestines (chit-lins, chitterlings).

Your organs will swell-up in size if many toxin's are taken into your system. The swelling is to aid the organ in gathering up more nutrients in an attempt to get the needed nourishments to the organ. This is why some people have large stomachs and bodies. These people need to get on a better nutrition system, so that their organs get the proper nutrition and go back to their normal size. This type of swelling will over stress an organ and lead to disease of that organ.

Giving Birth

Proper diet should be practiced months before giving birth and continued until the breast feeding period is over. During the actual conception of a child, and up until child birth, the parents diet, emotions, mental and spiritual state of being is being transmitted to the child.

Bowel Movements

Your body should secrete feces at lease once for each meal you eat per day. So if you eat three meals a day you should go to the rest room three times a day. And the feces should be solid but yet having a soft texture and not hard or slushy.

Teeth

Tooth decay is a condition found only in countries were processed foods or ate. Most toothpaste contain substances that or harmful to your teeth. Fluoride in tooth paste is very bad for your system. You should visit a health food store and purchase a paste which will not harm the teeth or better yet use water or non Aluminum Baking Soda to brush teeth and sea salt and water for a mouth wash. Bad breath can be a sign of illness in the body. Metal filling in you teeth will introduce mercury and other poisons into your system that will decrease the functions of your glands. Have them removed and replaced with a non metallic filling. Mercury fillings have been outlawed in other country's, and they are the cause of many nervous system disorders (disrupt the electrical energies of the body). Also they cause Alzheimer's disease. The plant Cilantro "Coriandre" can be eaten in your salads and will aid in the removal of mercury from your body. Ginkgo Biloba, a memory enhancing herb, is also a good treatment for Alzheimer's.

Care of the Vagina

Most of the tampons, douches, and douching liquids on the market contain chemical's that will harm the body (pollute it) and throw it out of balance. A woman should use natural products instead, such as vinegar and water douching liquids. A woman should not cover the vagina with non cotton materials such as nylon because these materials can prevent air flow to the vagina which can lead to yeast infection and other unwanted conditions.

Smoking

Tobacco smoke contains about 4,000 chemicals and at least 200 poisons. Why smoke you know that this will kill you eventually. And the smoke that a non-smoker inhales from a smoker's cigarette has higher amounts of these bad substances.

Marijuana

The smoking of Marijuana is bad for the majority of body functions and organs, including the brain and it can cause aging and early death. But, the eating of Marijuana (Hemp seeds or butter) is a good source of vitamins and minerals.

Memory Loss

Memory loss in some people is due to having too many toxins in the body (and Brain). The liver, if over loaded, can not remove all of the toxins. Also giving the brain more oxygen can increase memory and brain functioning. You increase oxygen flow by cleansing your body, exercise, keeping body pH on an alkaline non-acidic level (eat whole natural foods), breathing good sources of air (parks, away from smoke, gases etc…).

Pets, Animals

Various worms (parasites) can be transferred to humans from house pets. It is not good to have them in the home. You should give them an herbal parasite cleanser, bath them regularly and feed them a natural diet conducive to the animal type and wash hands and body after playing with them.

Bodily detection of illness and initial cleansing treatment

Illnesses of the organs can show up in the eyes and on the skin. Two signs that show up in the skin are a change in complexion or acne. Red veins in the eyes or a sign of illness in the body. Other places such as pain in sections of the feet or toes also fingers. Abnormal urine color (should be clear if system is clean) and change in feces texture (Hard, lumpy, slush-like). Hair breakage or loss of hair. Other mental sign's are: can't stay focused, easily irritated, mood swings, or loss of memory. If you have any of these ailments you should take an enema or eat prunes or other fruit or vegetable that will give you a good bowel movement. then you should squeeze a lemon or a half into a glass of water and drink it, this will clean your system out and help it to get back to its normal functions.

Vitamins and Minerals

It has been medically proven that black woman can produce vitamin "C" in their bodies if their diet is right.
Synthetic vitamins are not as good for you as the natural vitamins that you get from fruits vegetables, herbal tea's, and natural oils due to the fact that they have been processed.

Some of the vitamin mineral supplements found on the market today can cause ill effects such as head acne, kidney pain, bumps on face and other parts of the body, sleeplessness and an overly excited state. This is mainly due to what the substance were derived from and how it was processes. You should do some research in order to find good supplements such as wheat germ, flaxseed oil, virgin olive oil, Amino acids, Antioxins, Brewer's Yeast, grape seed extract and vitamin's "C" & "E".

The typical Western diet has 30% more fat in it than the African diet. This means that black people should lower their fat intake to insure good health (reduce or cut out all milk and meat products excluding some types of sea foods). Lack of the proper nutrients in your food will also reduce your sex drive.

Protein

Animal proteins are converted by the body into fats which can cause ill effects on your systems. Also animal proteins are not a complete source of proteins for the body, it can constipate you, and meat stays in your body to long and rots. Fresh whole grains, long grain rice, the herb nettles, nuts and seeds are a good source of proteins. Eating meats and processed foods causes a high acid content or pH in the body. This can lead to bad health conditions. A vegetarian diet causes a balanced alkaline level or pH in the body which results in better body functions and good health. In the Ancient African culture meat was only eaten when there were no fruits, nuts, grains or vegetable around to eat and at special ceremonies. Meat was not consumed on a daily basis.

A large amount of our eating habits or dictated to us by the company's that sell the food products, by way of advertisements, T.V., radio, signs, newspapers and is based on their company's profits, not your health. A Naturalist or Naturopathic Doctor, nutritionist, your personal research, and health food stores are a much better place to get information on which food types that you should consume.

Mixing of Food, pH and Digestion

You should try to eat different food types separately such as fruits, vegetables, grains, oils, starches, and meats (fish, foul (no chicken)). Eat each type of food at least 15 to 30 minutes apart to allow your body time to mix an adequate amounts of digestive fluids to the food, for proper digestion. So don't use oils on your salads. The mixing of foods types can also cause an imbalance pH reading in the body. Food must first have the proper amount of saliva mixed with it before it reaches the stomach, so chew your food well before swallowing it. The taste buds in your mouth senses the type of food, sends a signal to your brain then your brain tell your organs how much and what type of digestive fluid is required to digest the particular food.

An imbalance pH level will result in the body not having the proper alkaline or acid level which causes improper digestion of foods and the body and brain will not receive the right nutrition they need. The acids in soda's will throw you body's pH level off. A balance pH reading for the average person should be some where in the range of 4 - 7 (more alkaline pH is okay). A highly acidic pH reading (pH higher than 8) is bad for the body it will make your stomach very acidic causing acid reflux and other problems. Various herbs were eaten with foods in Ancient Egypt to aid a person in mixing the different food types so that they can be properly digested together in the body. This is where we got the modern day term called seasoning, but a lot of our modern day seasonings are not good for your system.

Allergy

I have also learned through experience that using herbs will also aid the body in digesting and eliminating the bad effects of allergy causing foods or substances. The uses of herbs have lessened the ill effects of my allergies a great deal. This is due to the fact that certain herbs cleanse your blood and organs. Also fasting and enemas will decrease the amount of allergy substances in your body giving you a degree of relief from the allergy symptoms. If you can't find the right herbs for your allergies, have a Naturalist or Naturopathic Doctor prescribe one of their herbal formula's for you. Allergy and Asthma sufferer's need to use Oxygen products (see below) and get rid of mucus causing substances in their diet such as milk (dairy products).

Stomach Worms

Stomach worms are the results of a poor diet. If a person has stomach worms when they eat, the worms eat their food and the person is living off the feces of the stomach worm. Proper nutrients, herbs, iron and proteins can prevent the occurrence of stomach worms.

Cooked Foods

Cooked foods are harder to digest and some or all of the nutrients (vitamins, minerals, enzymes) in the food are destroyed when the food is cooked. A good alternative is to steam or eat raw foods.

Processed Foods

Processed foods will cause ill effects on all the organs of the body, making it hard for them to adequately perform their job. Examples of processed food: White sugar, salt, white flour (bread), soda's, candy-bars, baking-soda ice-creams etc…

Vegetarian / Fruitatarian

Science has studied the body's digestive tract and has determined that the body requires a vegetarian diet to function properly and that a meat eater has a shorter life span than a Vegetarian / Fruitatarian. A Vegetarian or Fruitatarian diet contains all the nutrients required for proper body functions, yet a meat eater's diet doesn't. Watermelon is a good fruit to include in your diet, it has strong healing and cleansing powers, due to the fact that it contains hydrogen peroxide in its natural state.

A lot of people feel that they need to eat meat products to stay warm in the winter time. This is wrong. Your body heats up when you eat meat due to the fact that it is struggling to digest the meat. Your body is using up energy to process the meat. This energy could be used for other bodily functions. Vegetarian / Friutarian diet require less energy for digestion. Heart disease is mainly caused by bad dietary habits (eating the wrong foods) but fruits and vegetable are good foods for the heart.

Breads

If you are going to eat bread, eat breads made from un-processes wheats, and grains, with no processed white sugar or baking soda (contains Aluminum). Use non-aluminum baking soda. The carbohydrates in breads and pasta's turn into sugars and can cause tooth decay. Enriched flour is white in color, but the grain has color when it is in its natural state. These grains have been stripped of their nutrients during processing.

The Food Processing Industry

The Food Processing Industry makes money from selling you food. If they can make more money buy putting chemicals, synthetic foods, preservatives and poisons into the food you buy, I am sure that some of them will. The Government Agency's or here to protect your health (FDA, USDA) yet these company's generate billions of tax dollars for the government. Now will the Government put them out of business for selling you unhealthy food and will these Government officials not accept bribes from companies to past their product? You will have to watch out for your own health if you want to havegood health!

Cow's milk was meant for cows not human's. This milk contains all the hormones and other chemicals, such as Antibiotics, Pesticides, and Growth Hormones, which are shot into and feed to the cows. And most milks are deficient in fiber, iron, niacin and vitamins and contains a type of calcium that the body can not digest. Human require calcium from vegetables. In nature the mother stops giving milk when the child moves out of the infant stage. This is true for all animals and is why milk is not necessary in a non-infant or adults diet.

Here is a list of products that are bad for your health ice cream, candy bar's, chewing gum, products containing white sugar, milk, butter, cheese, yogurt, soda's, public drinking water (you should drink well water, spring water or distilled water). Margarine don't eat (much worse than butter) it is a plastic substance made by chemical companies. Snacks between meals slow down your digestive process and may cause constipation.

Herbs

Herbs should be taken in their natural state once the herb has been over heated it may change its chemical structure. So your tea's should not be over heated, just let them soak in warm water then drink them or take them straight in their natural form. If the body is full of processed bad foods and you are taking herbs, the herbs will be used up trying to correct the damage that the bad food did to your body, and none of the herbs will be used for normal body functions or healing. Examples of some herbs that can be consumed for good health, Cayenne pepper, Milk-thistle, dandelion root, Parsley, Alfalfa, Echinacea, Ginger and Goldenseal. Try to find loose herbs some of the packaged herbs or old and contain contaminants. African patients were instructed to use meditative (prayer) to clear their minds before they were given curative herbs.

Africa was once invaded by outsiders for it's herbs (healing power), but today Africa is raped of precious metals, jewels, people etc. There are other herbal products on the market such as cleaners, antibacterial air sprays, disinfectants, bug repellants, clothing detergents, body soaps, candies, drinks, mouth washes, deodorant, hair products, eye drops, lotions, herbs for your pets, herbal oils, etc.

Earth Minerals

These minerals can be obtained from the eating of plants, roots etc. If these mineral or left in the body for long periods of time it can cause the body to not process nutrients correctly and cause problems in your joints. Therefore these minerals can be removed from the body by the eating of fresh fruits. Remember that the nutrients in roots (or vegetables that grow underground) help to maintain the electrical systems of the body. They are used to activate various functions in the body, but should be removed from the body afterwards.

Body Chemistry

Black people's body chemistry is designed to process tropical plants (fruits, vegetables, herbs, seeds, nuts) for food. Examples of some of these plants are banana, cherry, watermelon, apricot, dates, pineapple, melons, figs, coconuts, lettuce, kiwi, grapes, papaya, apples, greens, pumpkin seeds, sunflower seeds, almonds etc…

Spiritual Oils

Sandalwood and Camphor are oils that activate the receiving and transmitting of spiritual energies in the body. Sandalwood is good for the pituitary gland.

Metals, Crystals

The body contains various metals (minerals). Metals, Crystals and Gems can transmit and receive various energy states. And these energy related properties were used in African healing practices example; Copper is good for your blood and Melanin in skin. Gold is good for intestines. Silver is good for electrical body currents, brain, and thyroid gland. Energies can be transmitted into the body's minerals (metals) by way of sunlight (life force energy), Color, or Music, to induce a particular effect upon the body or a specific organ.
Magnets and crystals can be used to reintroduce the correct energy state back into an ill part of the body.

Holistic Law

Always remember that Holistic law states that nothing just happens. Everything in the universe has a cause and effect related to it. Everything in the universe is linked together in some way or another.

Body Polarities

The top of the body is at a negative polarity and the bottom half is at a positive polarity. The right side of the body caries a positive polarity (gives energy) and the left side of the body carries a negative polarity (attracts energy). When looking at the whole body a woman is negative (magnetic - attracts energy) and a male is positive (electric - gives energy).

Music

Music sound waves (various frequencies of energy) inter the African body by way of the melanin in the body, such as ears (melanin), skin (melanin), eyes (melanin), and hair. Then this energy is used by the body for healing, general upkeep of the body, evoking different moods, or spiritual enlightenment and activation. Speaking or singing in various notes can send various vibrations or healing energies to and through the body. This is why we have junk food Rap music with and ill message. The music supplies you with good vibrational energies but the lyric hinders your thinking. Rap only talks of life in terms of sex and violence etc. This is mental brain washing not good for kids or weak adults. We need to listen to the old Soul, Jazz, and Reggae music were the music and lyrics present good vibrational energies to the mind and body.

Mind

Science has discovered that Black people use the right and mid sections of the brain when thinking. These sections of the brain are known to control such thoughts as love, spirituality, rational and creative thinking.

The pituitary glands, located in the brain region, are sensitive to the changes in the Earth magnetic fields. This gland receives electromagnetic energy from the Sun and Earth's electromagnetic energy cycle which in turn affects your thought patterns.

Spanking Children / Depression

In the past African children had various restrictions put on them when they did wrong. These restrictions were used to correct their behavior. A child's mental processing is hindered when the child is spanked or hit when he or she does wrong.

Some people become mentally depress at the same time of the year that a loved one died. This is due to the fact that their body since the energy that is present on that same time each year and it triggers the mind to remember the mood of that sad event. You can take the herb St. John's Wort to fight off this depressed state of mind.

Age

Ancient writings state that man had a natural pure diet and lived to be 400 to 1,000 years of age. Our non-holistic approach to life is what has shortened our life span, changed our thought processing and taken away our spirituality!

Computers Effects on Eye's

A good tip when working for long periods on a computer is to change your display to "High Contrast Black". This is when the writing is white and the background is black or some other dark color can be used. This will give a calmer feeling in the eye's while working on the computer and reduce stress on the eyes. Computers give off rays that or harmful to the body and eye's, so try to limit your use on them.

Men's Cycle

Men have a 28-29 day cycle, similar to the woman's cycle, were they experience mood swings due to the hormone changes that occur in their bodies during this period.
If a man has multiple ejaculations in a short period of time it will decrease the amounts of spinal fluid needed for proper physical well-being, thought processing and spiritual awareness.

Women / Men

Poor nutrition and drugs can lead to impotency in men and women. An ejaculation is a physical activity that should be physicaly, mentally and spiritually uplifting for both partners. In the same breath, a partnership or marriage should also be physically, mentally and spiritually uplifting for both partners. If it is not, problems will occur in the relationship. Black people must stop living by other cultures concepts of marriage (partnership), and use their own holistic approach. One of the major things to be learned from this approach is that a man must understand his feminine side and a woman must understand her masculine side, then the two or in a harmonious and balanced state. This will promote understating of each others mentally projected personnality.

Women

Menstruation is not a normal female process. It has been proven that woman on a vegetarian diet have much less blood loss during the menstruation period. High heel shoes can cause unnecessary stresses on a woman's back, hips, toes, ankles, knees and uterus.

We have all noticed the bond between the mother and the child. This natural bond is due to the fact that the Women brings Spirituality and Love to this world . These are the first and main things that should be taught to a child. Women have various qualities that make them a higher evolved being than their male counterpart, such an extra "X" chromosome which boost their immune systems, and many other qualities. I feel that a woman is given these qualities to assure that the human race does not die out and that there is always Spirituality and Love on this Earth. In some ancient writings it was said that women were stronger than men and fought in wars with the men. Women had more freedoms in ancient times than today. Men and women were equals in ancient times.

Breast

A woman's breast should not be strapped down and covered in nylon. The strapping down of the breast prevents the chest muscles from developing. Also nylon prevents the breast from receiving needed air. Cotton is the best material to be worn over the skin because it lets the skin breath.

Nature

Over the years nature has deteriorated to a certain degree. This lowering from its natural state is due to the pollution (water, food and air), lower mental thoughts, and less spirituality. This loss has resulted in a lower quality of food, minerals, vitamins, vegetation, human's etc. We must return to a holistic way of life if we want nature to return to its proper state. We must stop trying to force nature to adhere to our rules and start abiding by the laws of nature. Don't eat, think or do what nature did not intend for you to do. We are presently living against nature and this is why our life span is not as long as it was in ancient times 150 or more years of age. We or contracting all types of diseases. We

have lost the understanding of the Spiritual Powers that were given to us by the Creator (we have little to no Spirituality in our lives).
There exist a Law in nature called, "Gia's Revenge", that says if you go against nature then nature will destroy you for you are a part of nature, you are not higher than nature and shall abide by the laws of nature.

Sex

Poor sex drive in men and women and large losses of blood during a womans monthly cycle can be a direct result of poor diet. Some sexual diseases are only present when the body is out of balance such as when the diet or mental faculties or out of balance. We should only have sex during the natural mating seasons.

Having to much sex can shorten the life span and weakens the sexual organs, which can result in a diseased organ. During sexual intercourse the body loses required energies need for it to function. Due to changes in hormone levels, excessive sex decreases the minds ability to function. In the African culture sexual intercourse only happened during mating seasons. Sexual intercourse was for the creation of offspring only and was not a recreational activity as we use it today. Sex should be performed in the day light hours, when the body is at its highest energy state, not at night. Excessive sex has been brought on by society's poor standards and morals, hormones in the meat, and other non-natural reasons. A poor quality of sperm from the male can lead to a miscarriage or a weakening of the offspring's health. Always remember that the physical, mental and spiritual state of the parents during intercourse is passed on to the child so be sure that your partner is of a high physical mental and spiritual state of being.

Sexual Perversion \ Homosexuality

The Creator made man and woman so that they would mate and keep the race going and enhance each others state of being. For this reason and others, homosexuality goes against the Laws of the Creator. When sperm and feces inter the body through anal sex the immune system is weakened.

Herpes

Herpes is just the bodies attempt to rid itself of waste materials. Good body cleansing and proper diet will eliminate herpes. In African science organs function in groups such as the testicles and ovaries with the kidneys pineal and pituitary glands. So remember when one organ is weakened it will soon weaken another organ causing more stress on the body.

Antibiotics

Antibiotics will lower your immune systems functions, which leads to a weaker body that can't fight off disease at its normal capacity. So do your best not to take antibiotics. Antibiotic's or put in cows and other animals food. You eat these drugs when you eat the meat and milk of the cow or other animal.

Ritalin

The drug Ritalin disrupts the normal functions of the mind (drive a person crazy), because it disrupts the nervous system.

Sleep

A person should always get the proper amount of rest each day. The average person requires at least six to eight hours a day. When you are sleep you give the brain and body more time and energy to perform its natural functions, one of which is healing. Try to take napes when you are ill. You should awake with the Sun and go to sleep with the Moon because your body follows nature's cycles. The sleeping state is also a spiritual state of existence, when you sleep the mind forms a stronger link between the body, mind and spirit. The proper sleeping position is to lay on the right side and this will promote proper breathing during your sleep.

Jewelry

The wearing of jewelry can introduce various metals into your body through the skin, stop wearing or only wear on special occasions. "Especially Cheap Jewelry" Metals and other substances can accumulate in the body and lower the function of various organs.

Lemons

Lemons should be eaten due to the fact that they aid in cleansing the body, it balances the body's alkalinity, and provides the body with needed enzymes. Also it puts the body back into its correct electrical state (Proper Frequency). Eat a lemon (or half) if you suffer from joint pains such as Arthritis or the pain you get after exercising and from the joint pain when it rains. The lemon will balance out the electrical state in the joints and the pain will go away. Also the Herbs Evening Primrose, Nettles and Boswellia are good for arthritis and joint pain. Eat lemon, if you suffer from any form of cancer, because the lemon will aid in re-balancing the electrical part of the body. Example: I have an old knee injury that plagues me from time to time. One day the knee was hurting very bad. I ate half of a lemon. After about one minutes my knee had stopped hurting.

Garden

Start your own garden in your yard or indoors. I did my 1st garden and I could not believe how easy it was. All I did was to plant them, water them, and then eat them. I ate watermelon, peas, and two types of beans, lettuce, and spinach from my garden. Fresh foods are best for your body. Fresh natural foods contain all the nutrients in their natural state, which the body needs.

Petroleum Jelly

Petroleum means oil (like the oil and gas you use in your car) I don't recommend using this on your skin as a moisturizer because your body will ingest it through the skin.

African Yoga

The head stand (head on floor or pillow, hands out to side on floor) or hanging upside down is an African Yoga position that stimulates the bodies elimination systems. It will aid the body in riding itself of toxins and waste. And their or many other yoga positions that you can use in your daily exercise routine.

Light Bulbs

Use full spectrum light bulbs in your home. They last longer and are more comfortable to the eye. These light bulbs were designed to simulate the light spectrum of sunlight and are better for you and your indoor plants.

Transmutation

The Laws of transmutation states that higher levels of energy can alter the structure of lower forms of energy and this is why humans and plants, if they or in good health can create the nutrients they need by changing one element into another required element. Also this is why the Sun's Energy can heal you. You use the energy from the sun which is stored in your body to transmutate one substance into another.

Colonic Irrigation

A colonic irrigation will take out all the waste materials that have accumulated in the colon and intestine due to a bad diet and drugs. This process is similar to the water bottle enema; a water and herbal solution is feed in through the anus in order to expel the accumulated waste.

Vaccination Shots

Vaccination Shots contain substances that will decrease the effects of your immune system, and some of them can cause extreme illnesses. So ask for forms to fill out that will exempt you or your child from taking any kinds of vaccination shots.

Diet

In this modern society there are over 300,000 types of edible plants and fruits but, approximately 59 are all that is used for food, something is wrong with this system. Yet Ancient Africans had over 200 types of edible plants and fruits in their diet.

Constipation / Bodily Germs and Bacteria

Research has shown that constipation is one of the main causes of disease, and the altering of the germs and bacteria that live in the body is another. Germs and bacteria have a natural balance in the human body that can be altered by the use of drugs and a bad diet.

High Blood Pressure / Joint Pain

If you are taking high blood pressure medicine get off this medication. It only shortens your life span. You should be taking Harthornberry (herb), omega-3 fatty acids, CoQ10(C0-enzyme 10). Also if you have joint pains, MSM Sulfur is the best thing for this and not drugs, also lemon juice. Go see a Naturopathic or Naturalist Doctor for the best natural cures for high blood pressure. High blood pressure is decreasing your life span by speeding up the natural rhythms and flows of the body, like a car being driven constantly at 100 miles per hour, some parts (organs) will soon fail.

One major contributor to high blood pressure is the consumption of caffeine (carbonated beverages, coffee, tea's), and don't use decaffeinated products cause they may contain chemicals that harm the body. Caffeine interferes with the function of the glands and kidneys.

African Priest

African Priest in ancient times were doctors, astronomers, agriculturist, chemist, psychologist, mathematicians, astrologist, engineers, sociologist, herbalist etc… And each had to study all the above areas of knowledge and more, so that their teachings would be holistic.

Prescription Drugs

If you eat grapefruits while on prescription drugs the grapefruit may increase (amplify) the effects of the drugs.

Modern medicine is base on the physical and chemical make up of a white male, all others shall be mis-diagnosed and wrongly treated to a certain degree. Also modern medicine tells you that herbs are bad for you in an attempt to stop you from growing them and treating yourself. Instead you go and buy these harmful prescription drugs.

Don't Always believe the Label

Just because the label says one thing check the ingredients to see if it actually is that product or a mixture of non-food substances that you would rather not eat.
Ingredients labels on products: the first is the largest amount contained in the product; the last is the least amount. Health food labels will show you how the labels should read, large amounts of main ingredient and no preservatives chemicals or dyes etc.

Animal Organs

Animal organs should not be eaten by humans they contain substances that are not good for your health.
Example; the liver is a waste filled gland and chitterlings are a waste (feces) filled organ (intestines), that should not be eaten.

Body Structure and Makeup

Don't try to change your natural body structure. If your bone structure is small, medium or large. Accept your beautiful structure and don't over or under eat, take drugs, are get mentally depressed about it. Because the truth of the matter is that all people come in different sizes shapes and colors, variety is the spice of life, and no shape size or color is better. All you can do is keep that body as healthy as you can and all will love you for it.

Parasites / Cancer

A parasite is a harmful organism that lives inside your body and feeds off the body. Doctor's have stated that parasites in your body and Propyl alcohol (a solvent) have been the cause of some cancers. Herbs and oils can be used to rid your body of parasites. Herbs such as Black Walnut and Worm Wood can be used to rid the body of parasites. Propyl alcohol (may not be on label) is found in the following list of items and should not be ingested or put on your body: shampoo's, mousse, cosmetics, mouth wash, shaving supplies, rubbing alcohol, white sugar, hair sprays, carbonated drinks. Also parasites plus the solvent benzene have been said to be a cause of disease. Benzene and propyl acohol gets into your bones and cells and decreases the effectiveness of your immune system. Other remedies for parasites or as follows: lemon, caster oil, worm wood, walnut hulls, vinegar, Organic sulfur (MSM), pine needles, and garlic. Also there are herbal parasite cleanser formulas on the market. Eating white processed sugar contribute to parasites in the body. The Shiitake mushroom is good for curing cancer and is an immune system booster. Also the Miatake mushroom is an immune system booster.

Organic Sulfur (MSM)

MSM sulfur helps to repair all cells in your body, it aids in the growth of hair and nails and cleanses the body.

Detergents / Dish Washing Liquids

Some cleansers contain PCB's and other harmful chemicals try to use a coconut or lemon based cleaner from a health store.

Rolled Oats

Oats are a good food to eat (contains Fiber, Protein and Iron), but the metal nickel, has been found in instant or one minute oats, so by the whole oats instead. Also try health food store brands their most likely priced the same or cheaper and is probably fresher.

Naturalist or Naturopathic Doctors (N.D.)

This type of doctor uses naturally occurring foods, herbs and substances to cure disease and maintain good health. Unlike medical doctors (M.D.'s) who use unnatural substances to treat disease. These unnatural substances have many side effects and cause other illnesses. Your body operates on the chemistry of nature because it is part of nature and not off man-made chemicals (prescription drugs). So you should use herbs to heal cure and maintain your body because herbs or also part of nature. A naturalist doctor try's to prevent illnesses before they occur, and to build the bodies systems up to their highest levels. They state that if the body is in good health it will heal and repair it's self of all illnesses, damage or disease. They can prescribe herbal formulas and natural foods that you need to consume for good health. They can tell you all the different foods you need to eat to maintain a balanced supply of nutrients (vitamins, minerals etc.) in your body. Many people have turned to the Naturalist doctors when the Medical doctors could not help them and were cured. Some people think that herbs are harmful to your health. This is not true. I feel that it is just propaganda created to steer people away from the Naturalist doctors. Example: I took five different herbal formulas at the same time which were made from a total of

96 different raw unprocessed herbs. And the only effects I got from these herbs were that my energy and circulation increased, my skin and hair looked great, and I felt great. The formulas that I took were as listed: bone muscle and tendon, memory concentration and circulation, lungs and respiratory, sugar balance, thyroid and a body cleansing formula.

Raw Seeds

Unsalted uncooked pumpkin seeds are rich in minerals including zinc and reduce risk of cancer and disease. Sunflower and Hemp Seeds are high in vitamins and minerals. Sunflower and pumpkin seeds contained needed Omega Essential Fatty-Acids which aid in the maintenance of the cells in the body and strengthening the immune system.

Meat Eaters

Certain animals should never be eaten cause their purpose in life is to rid the Earth or sea's of waste materials (they eat waste, garbage, feces). Some of these animals or as listed: pig, chicken, catfish, shrimp, crabs, lobsters. If I could put a label on the pig I would put the poisonous cross bones symbol on it. Also pork can be found in various medications such as insulin, suppositories, antacids, baby formula's etc. Eating meat, preservatives, chemicals and the other things that are added to the foods that you consume will decreases a persons ability to control his bodily functions and metal emotions.

Religious Passages

"and the leaves of the trees were for the healing of the nations", "and the fruit thereof shall be for meat, and the leaf there of for medicine", " it is good neither to eat flesh or drink wine", " my people are gone into captivity, because they have no knowledge"

AIDS

Former employees, stated that in 1969 the Dept. of Defense asked for and got money to produce the Aids virus (Check library of congress for this fact). Reports say that the Small-Pox Vaccination was given to people all around the world and it was laced with the Aids virus. Some say a different measles vaccination is given to the people in the ghetto's, and is 1st given to people on Welfare. This vaccination program is headed by the " CDC " Center for Disease Control which is the same group that injected and let the Disease Syphilis run rampant in the bodies of a group of black males, just so they could see what damage the decease would do to the body.

The American Indian and the Aborigine people of Australia were all wiped out (lowered to a very low population total) by disease warfare. This same type of disease warfare was used on the African people of South Africa. The White

invaders used all types of diseases on the Black people their but it failed. South Africa was later taken over by the White invaders after they gave the African Priest money and power, to teach the people a ritual that involved the burning of all crops and live-stock. The people then went into a state of starvation and then the Whites took over South Africa. All the above or forms of population control also cigarettes, drugs, and alcohol ect… or also forms of control.
A Spermicid containing the chemical called Nonoxynol can be used in sexual intercourse and it will kill the aids virus on contact. Also there are condoms (Trojan) and Lubricants (KY-Jel) that contain this virus killing chemical. Once you raise your bodies frequency, vibration, or life force energy to a higher level diseases like AIDS and viruses can no longer exist in your body.

A positive HIV Test does not mean that a person will contract AIDS. It means that the person's bodily defense system has boosted itself to a higher level so that it can fight off any diseases that the body may contract. Some people get a positive test back and feel that they have AIDS and the mental stress destroys their body's defense system and they get ill from any and even the weakest of diseases.

History shows that African's and other Non-White peoples had little to no disease until they came into contact with Whites. This is when diseases such as measles, small pox, mental illness, syphilis, the plague and other disease's got into the systems(body) of Non-White peoples, causing large scale sicknesses and deaths. The Diseases of Whites was caused by their unhealthy lifestyle, lack of melanin and a refusal to have a holistic approach to life.

Teaching Children

We must stop leaving it up to the schools and churches to teach or children physical, mental and spiritual health. We are the parents of the child and their 1st source of information and guidance. Teach them the truths found in these writings.

A large Number of Black Children all around the Globe are being kidnapped, killed and lamed so that their organs and bodily fluid can be used in formula's that will aid an older person in having more vitality. Also these children and or their body parts are being used in various types of experiments, so watch your children and watch out for the underhanded techniques and lie's that or used to gain access to your child or their body parts, fluids ect…

Other Health Tips

* A person can balance the bodily energies by placing the left hand approximately one inch above the top of the head and the right hand over the naval. This can be done twice a day morning and night or when you have a headache or feel ill.

* Studies show that aprox. 6 thousand billion pages of Info. can be stored in the Brain. Use the storage space for knowledge that can aid you in every day living not to memorize soap opera's and sports events.
* Spend some time every day with your mind (spend time alone, think beautiful, educational and spiritual thoughts.
* Don't be a person of words but of actions.
* This is a male oriented society and we must understand how to put the femininity back into it.
* Stop watching unrealistic things on TV and read a book on nutrition, spirituality etc...
* Remember that your existence centers around mind (your mental state). So read books that up lift your mental state.
* Our emotions and feelings or tied to our hormones and brain functions (feelings) which or in turn tied to our diets. Now if the diet is off then the emotions and attitude is off also (sad, mad, easily upset. Example: Women monthly cycle, some women get very moody due to the hormone change in their body and they have a different attitude than normal. But Health professionals say that a woman does not need to have a monthly cycle if she eats right and exercises. And long ago Black African women did not have a monthly cycle. The better you eat and exercise the lesser the amount of fluid discharged in your monthly cycle. Also when kids and adults eat the sugars in candy they get hyper and bad tempered.
* Take a blood purifier, cleanser each day. dandelion root, saspirilla burdock, goldenseal, enchineachia. Alternate your usage of the above blood cleansers.
* Dandelion root is good for your pineal gland (third eye).
* The scientist are searching for that which makes the black man/woman so strong, it is relates to your melanin and is called the phebanache principle of melanin energy.
* By way of mental thought energy black people can make physical energy.
* White people only produce a little melanin in their bodies, this is due to pineal gland calcification.
* Chem = black = melanin, chemistry = study of melanin.
* On the white man's arrival to America they described the Indian's as to having thick lips, woolly hair and black skin. This is a description of the Black African woman/man.
* Their is no written history of any black man ever selling another black man, in a slavery type of system.
* 3 Table spoons of sugar = 28ft of sugar cane, to much for the human body.
* Aspirin lowers blood flow to the sexual organs.
* Starches (rice, potatoes) digest well with vegetables.
* Calcium Phosphate = good calcium for the body to ingest
* In the brain is where the pineal gland, black dot or Third-Eye is located. It is larger in black people, this part of your brain connects you to all in the universe.
* Bumps on the forehead is a sign that intestine or probably clogged (constipation).
* Bags under the eyes equals kidney problems.

* Eyes watery kidney problems, eyes yellow liver problems.
* Calluses on feet tells you what is wrong in your body, see a reflexology chart for more info.
* There or 22 types of Iron, to be sure you are getting the right type, eat the whole foods that contain iron, beets etc.
* Chewing gum has cancer causing agents in it and many other bad things in it, like petroleum products.
* Beers, and malt liquor have petroleum, lead and alcohol's in them.
* The bodies first warning signs are of the feminine principle (soft, nurturing) Example: The soft voice in your head that says that the food you ate might make you sick, later the masculine comes in when you get that bad ache in your gut and run to the restroom. Today's medical establishments only uses the masculine principle which is usually after the illness has progressed to for.
* Black people in America don't eat African foods we eat Chinese, Italian, white (European) etc…
* Feminine = sense, feel, think then balance it. you should talk to a woman in a feel it type of way.
* Masculine = sense, think, feel, then balance it. you should talk to a man in a think it type of way.
* George Washington Carver (Black man) was a modern day Alchemist.
* The hormones in the beef chicken and fish are the cause of kids going through puberty to fast. Girls getting breast and period two soon.
* You should season food after you cook it. You should steam vegetables.
* In nature bright colors are masculine colors (red, orange, yellow). Blue, purple green are feminine.
* Black woman have a high decease and death rate than any other races, cause the medical establishment treats all on a white male standard, leaving out the female principle and the black persons melanated body type.
* Herbs: Catnip, St.-Johns Wort, Feverfew, Chamomile in juice or water will stop a child from being over-active. Also St-Johns Wort can be used for cleansing the liver, take a dose each day.
* Garlic and Ginger is good for your intestines.
* Cayenne pepper, watermelon, beets or good for the digestive organs of the body.
* Wheatgrass and Spirulina for colon up keep.
* We should all wear African hair styles that promote a healthy head of hair and body. Such as Braids, Twist, Afro's, Locks. What you put on your hair and scalp goes into your body. So use eatable products such as fruit and vegetable juices on the hair.

African History and Contributions to the World

We must first understand that all Black people around the world are Africans. We then must learn of the contributions that our African Ancestors have made to the world. Due to the fact that this knowledge is rightfully yours and the truth of the matter is that this knowledge is still within you. It was pasted through the genetics of your great grand parents (African Egyptians) on to you at birth. Now is the time to activate these knowledge centers in the brain and pull from your great oasis of knowledge (Brain, and Spirit).

In an attempt to gain proof of the above fact please note in your family how certain people act, think, look and have the same interest ect... as some older member of the family, whom they may or may not have had contact with. Example; I saw my grandfather once and knew very little about his life. He moved away when his kids were very young. He and one of my uncle's and I are all tall unlike the rest of the family. My grandfather was an Electrical Engineer in the army, my uncle was an Electrical Specialist in the army and I am an Electrical Engineer. I did not know until well after gaining my degree that my grand father was and Electrical Engineer in the army and he left when my uncle was around five years old. And my uncle joined the army for a 20 year stay, before I was born. I feel that we inherited the same interest as my grandfather from his genetics. Also my grandmother dreamed things often that came true, and now my mother did the same. I feel this visionary state or gift was past on from mother to daughter through their genetics. In this same way our ancient african knowledge is within us all.

Knowledge of Self

We must gain knowledge of self (our African History), or as written in Ancient Egyptian Temples "Know Thyself". The Ancient Black African Egyptians developed a very complex social, system, called the Maathian Creed (Mystery System), which was also the first and oldest system based on the existence of the Creator (God) and what is the purpose of life.

This system brought fourth to the world the first and highest ever reached levels of science, religion, medicine, philosophy, social systems, astrology, art, music, math, alchemist, hermetics (philosophy), hieroglyphics (reading, writing, alphabets), geometry, numerology, engineering, ethics, astronomy, botany, herbologist, educational systems, zoology, metaphysics, mortuary science, the calendar, yoga, karate, physics, poetry, military science, law, magic and many other highly intellectual subject matter. Which were the makings of the Black Egyptian civilization.

And all of this knowledge was based on truth and was past on by way of the priest to all the people upon this planet in an attempt to get all of man-kind on one common mental physical and spiritual state. Which would bring forth peace and harmony to all and raise the conscious level of man-kind to its highest level. Also the Black Egyptian Priest could not accept money in return for their services to the public. For hundreds of years man-kind has been lead to believe that the Greeks and Romans brought the above intellectual knowledge systems to the world which belong to the Ancient Black African Egyptian people. Thousand of Ancient African artifacts are stored away in British, American and other Museums around the world, in an attempt to hide the high level of knowledge and great advancements of the African people.

We must denounce all Greek lettered fraternities and sororities from our Black colleges and culture. It was put there only to brain wash you into a lower mental state than that of White people. They sould be African named human upliftment groups instead. Please note that our modern western society promotes a negative way of thinking, on the TV, radio, newspapers, schools, churches and other media for which these false statements can be projected to all people. Malcolm-X once said "that just because Europeans or the dominant race, this does not mean that they or superior". This statement mean that just because a particular group of people presents the elusion of being the physical ruling power at that time, does not mean that they have a higher social structure or higher physical mental or spiritual state of being than that of other groups of people. We must erase our old mind set which was given to use and not produced from our own mental conclusions (minds and culture) but that which was given to us.

Every person is born more so as a perfect being but that which you input into a persons brain is what corrupts us all, because we have inputted untruths instead of truths. This system tells us that being a Black African, dark-skinned, braids, locks, thick lips, round buttocks is wrong, but to be European is right. We need to get back to our cultural ways and produce a proper mental state in our people. We must stop brain washing our children and society by teaching non-African ways which go against our hold physical mental and spiritual state of being. When you give your physical, mental and spiritual energy to Non-African causes you destroy all which is African and in return destroy your self.

This western society falsely credits Roman and Greek people, such as Aristotle, Plato, Pythagoras as the creators of the Black Egyptian Philosophies and other intellectual works. When you trace these persons history back it takes you back to the Egyptian Schools were they were taught. Also their life history is very vague as to how they progressed up to be such a knowledgeable level. Some of these persons were accredited to have written far more books than they could have written in a life time. During the time period that these books should have been written by the Roman and Greeks, they had many internal wars going on within their countries which would have slowed progress of all kinds in those countries, including the writing of books. When you study Greek and Roman's intellectual writings you find out that they or very similar to that of the Egyptian's intellectual writings. But history proofs that the Egyptians existed long before the Greeks and the Romans and they had an intellectually higher level of Society than that of the Greeks and Romans.

Mystery System

The African Egyptian Mystery System Schools of ancient times were the oldest and most widely dispersed schooling systems. It always did and still carries the belief in one God only, the Creator. It had sub-schools in Rome, Greece, China, Mexico, North America, Japan, Arabia, Malaysia and many other places, which carried out its teaching all over the world. The fact that there exist pyramids all over the globe is proof that the Egyptian creators of the pyramids had spread their knowledge all over the world. The Mystery system temples were all adorn with markings denoting the Zodiac and Celestial cycles of the planet and stars. These markings were symbolic of the connection between all things in the Universe. The Mystery System teachings consisted of many intellectual levels yet the Roman and Greeks were not allowed to participate in any knowledge above the third degree, due to the fact of their uncivilized nature (mental state of being).

Masonic Lodges, Freemasonry

Freemasonry was started by the Black Egyptians long before the modern day freemasonry groups and long before the White man invaded Africa. The original freemasonry groups followed the Maathian Creed Laws (Laws of Maat) and some of these same original masonic groups exist today all around the Globe. The modern day Masonic Lodges (Mason's) are copies of the Ancient African Egyptian Mystery Systems. These Masonic lodges may or may not up-hold the same teaching of the Ancient Egyptian Temples. It is left up to your discretion to determine if the teachings of a particular lodge are the same as that of the Primary Mystery System Schools of Egypt. Some of these lodges are not teaching for the uplifting of mankind. They are only concerned with the up-lifting of their lodge members. So a person must use his/her God given skill of judgment to determine which group is right for you.

Down Fall of the Egyptian Mystery System

History States that Egypt had the highest level of civilization upon this planet for thousands of years. Some say that this Egyptian society existed 300,000 to 600,000 years ago. The initial downfall of Egyptian society began when the Black Egyptian leaders began to feel that they were as powerful as the Creator (God). They did not have control of their ego. This sparked off disagreements and caused the separation of the Egyptian empire into many small groups. The African Egyptian's had fought off many invaders for thousands and thousands of years before this time of turmoil. Now they were invaded by many other groups such as the Persians. The Roman/Greeks lead by Alexander the Great were the last of these invaders.

This time period approximately 6,000 years ago marks the end of the Egyptian Empire. Later, during the Roman/Greek rule of Egypt the social structure started to deteriorate at a fast rate. During this time period the Roman/Greeks started to change the Egyptian Divinities to Asiatic (White, European peoples) names, faces and philosophies. Note: When a Group of People (Romans) concur another group of people(Egyptian) the concurring group forces the other groups people to take their identity. Why did the Romans not follow this rule? They instead took the identity of the Egyptians. I feel that they did this because they knew that in that time period and all around the world the Egyptian name carried much moor weight than the Roman name. So they wanted to be seen as the highest culture of people, but they were not.

A system of mental destruction was inserted into the African social structure in this time of slavery. And this system was based on color of skin, hair texture, living quarters, heights and many others differences of the slaves. This system created hatred among the slave and cause them to hate one another. It was said that this system would fuel itself and would keep the Black slaves fighting among themselves and they would never know who the real enemy (oppressor) was. This state of mind is still so vivid in our b Black culture and must be erased so that the Black man can move to a higher mental state.

First Spiritual Teachings / Christian Era

The original spiritual teachings of the Isis and Osiris Stories (Asar and Auset) of the Egyptian Mystery System were altered by the Roman/Greeks invaders. (Osiris was also called The Lord of the Perfect Black). During the time of the Roman Rule of Egypt a decree was made by the Roman/Greeks that they have the Egyptian people (have them enslaved) but we don't have their religion. The Egyptian people still practiced their religion (way of life system) while they were enslaved under Roman /Greek rule. And this is why the Roman/Greek Christian religion era as we know it today began. The Roman/Greek rulers took the Black Egyptian's Isis and Osiris religious (way of life system) stories and rewrote them in an attempt to brain wash the people into a slave mentality and to replace the African leadership figures with that of Greek/Roman (White) leadership figures, in an attempt to erase the African Egyptian's way of life (spiritual and social) systems. And this is when and why the Christian Bible as we know it today was written by the Greek/Romans people. This is the same Bible used in the majority of all the churches in America such as Roman Catholic, Christian, Methodist, Jehovah-Witness, and many other churches. Some of the churches that don't use this Greek/Roman Bible are the Buddhism, Muslims and other churches.

We must note also that some of the books of the Bible have been left out of the Bible such as the book of Enoch. We must refer to the Dead Sea Scrolls, Nahamati, Tebetian and other Writings for more info on these lost books of the Bible. The Greek/Roman rulers were unable to read the spiritual Isis and Osiris stories so they forced some of the Egyptian Priest whom which did not leave the area when Egypt came under Greek/Roman rule, to aid them in the writing of the Bible. From this I have derived that if you are of a higher spiritual conscious (mental) state then you will understand the Bible as the Egyptian Priest wanted you to. But if you do not poses a high spiritual conscious state, at the time of your reading of the Bible, then you will be enslaved and mislead by the Bible as the Roman/Greeks intend it to be used. Most of use or not at this higher spiritual state of being and that is why we are being fooled today. Therefore the Bible is a confusing conglomeration of truths and lies and it is up to the reader to differentiate between the two. There exist many other spiritual writings as listed above that you can use to compare to the Roman/Greek Bible. They should be reviewed and compared to the Roman/Greek Bible so that you can make a good personal choice of spiritual guidance.

If you trace back all spiritual writings, you will find out that the Isis and Osis stories or the oldest and first spiritual writings, and all others were derived from this initial African Spiritual Masterpieces. These writings taught that if you base your life on the obtainment of truths and then the following of these truths, not untruths, then you will reach the highest level of spirituality known to mankind. If you have a calm metal state and think from the heart (love for self and mankind) then you can use the abilities that the creator gave to us all, of knowing what is right and what is wrong. We must all realize that all books were written by mankind and or subject to era. Any group of people when writing their religious and other books can write what they like into these books. And all we have to aid us in the understanding of these books and spirituality is our God given ability to think from the heart (differentiate between a truth and an untruth).

We don't need a book, but we can use a good book to aid us. I am sure that at birth the All Mighty Creator(God) gave each man all that he needs to move her/his self to the highest levels of spiritual understanding (his/her body, mind, and spirit). Read on for more proofs of the above statements.

Black people in America or like orphans we don't realize that our ancestor were the creator's of the first religious systems for which all present day religion's were derived from. We say that all people have a spirit self, but do we ever try to use this spirit-self, for it is more powerful than the human self. We must link our minds to the physical and the spiritual self so that we can use all the powers that the Creator has instilled in us all.

There were White groups of people all throughout time whom practiced the African Maathean Creed Religious system also. And these people were prosecuted by the Roman Catholic's and Political Powers due to the fact that they did not follow the Roman Catholics Christian Religious beliefs.

Mission of Christianity

When the Greek/Roman people initiated the start of the Christian era (not to be confused with the Coptic Christian Era) their aim was to have it replace the old world religion which was the African Egyptian mystery system teachings. The Egyptians sent priest out to other lands to convince and teach the message of truth contained in the Isis and Osiris spiritual teachings. But during the Roman/Greek occupation of Egypt, the Roman/Greeks sent missionaries to other lands in an attempt to conquer the lands and force their Christian religion onto the people of those lands by way of force or trickery. These methods are still being used by today's leaders to control peoples and their land and resources.

Trinity

In the modern day Roman/Greek Bible the Trinity is represented as the Father the Son and the Holy Spirit. I do not agree with this statement. In this context the Trinity represents the act of Creation, which is the Mother the Father and the Child, which is the same as the African Egyptian spiritual Trinity of Isis (Mother), Osiris (Father), and Horus (Child). The Mother (-) and the Father (+) unites in the creation of Child (+) or (-). Another creation trinity is that of the Sun, Moon and the Earth. The Sun and Moon Sustains life on Earth. They act as the Earths parents creating and sustaining life on earth. The moon initiates the growth process in all vegetation and it has a controlling affect on the waters of the Earth. and the Sun brings forth the life sustaining energy to all living things upon the Earth. Just to name a few reasons why the Moon and the Sun exits. Please note that God is the Supreme Creator therefore God is the Mother (-) and the Father (+) of all things. There exist other trinities also such as the three states of Creation: Physical, Mental and Spiritual. Another Trinity is the three stars in the Orion Constellation, which the three pyramids of Giza are positioned after.

Loss of Knowledge

The Greek/Roman people were unable to decipher the majority of the vast amounts of spiritual and intellectual information that they had obtained from the African Egyptian Mystery System writings. It was also said that they burned hundreds of the Egyptian books stored in the Egyptian Mystery System Temples and Library's such as the famous Library's of Alexandria and Menephtheion. And many of the other books or in European Libraries or locked away for only a select few people to view them.

The Egyptian Priest-Hood

An Egyptian priest (Shaman) education took approximately 50yrs to complete (and was taught in a holistic manner) and progressed through many degrees of learning for which the Greeks priest had only been taught up to the 3rd degree. And only Black African's were taught in the higher degree's. The Egypt Priesthood existed a long time before what the western history books tell you. The Egyptologists tell you that the Egyptian society only existed back to about ten thousand years ago. But other historians, ruins, and archeologist say Egypt existed 50, 100 to 10,000 thousand years ago. Moses in the Bible was an initiate of the African Egyptian mystery system. An in the Ancient times the Egyptian had the highest level of culture and many people from all over the world came to Egypt to be taught at Egyptian mystery system schools.

After the Roman/Greek Invasion of Egypt, many of the Egyptian priests fled to other lands and set up the spiritual teachings of the Egyptian mystery system in these lands. One such group was the Moor's whom which fled to Spain and reestablish the African teaching there.

The invaders (Greek/Romans) claimed that they were the authors of the Mystery system books. When the true authors were the Black Egyptian Priest. And they have continue this practice up until the present time. An the books that they or claiming or on various subject matter such as spirituality, science, Metaphysic, Astrology, Mathematics, Alchemy and many other subjects. Their were different educational avenues that an Egyptian Priest could take and depending on the avenue he was undertaking, she / he had to master one or many of the many books of Hermes, which held that particular subject matter of choice.

Before they took their major courses of study they were taught the basic Arts and Virtues. Also they learned secret languages and writing techniques that only the Egyptian priest understood. From their teaching the priest obtained abilities such as hypnosis, mental levitation and prophecy telling, from which people gave them the title of Witches and Warlocks whom which practiced Magic. This can be known from the Egyptian head gear worn by Merlin The Magicians. The magician wore a cone shaped hat with stars and other astral bodies on it symbolizing the Egyptian style of head gear and the stars and astral bodies representing the practice of Black Egyptian Astrology. The Magical abilities that the priest displayed were the highest order of knowledge, of the laws of nature. The term Witches, Warlocks and Magic were given a negative connotation by the Greek/Roman's in order to steer the masses away from the Ancient African Mystery teachings. So that their highest Physical Mental and Spiritual levels of knowledge would not be obtained by the descendants of Africa or any other group that was not of the same mind-set as the Greek/Roman Empire.

The Egyptian Priest also were the author's of "The Book of Coming Forth by Day and by Night" ("The Book of the Dead"), "The 42 Law's of Maat" and "The Kybalion" which are all teachings on how to obtain salvation for the soul (spirit self) while on Earth. Please note that the Priest were women and men. Before the downward spiral of the Egyptian society. The Priest would memorize all required information in their schooling. I assume this ability was lost as society started to decline.

The Knowledge Within You

The African American and all other African descendants around the world must give up their feelings of inferiority and return to a higher state of being as their Egyptian ancestors had obtained. We must realize that all this knowledge of the mystery system was past on to us through our genetics, if only we would put our minds in the correct mental state to extract and use the knowledge within us all. The present economic system was created to keep one group of people in power and to stop others from advancing. We must realize that the Creator (God), not the present system of things, is the highest power in this universe.

Christianity's Hold On The Black Man

We must first realize that for thousands of years we have been forced and tricked into erasing our old Black Egyptian way of life system and to follow the European Christian way of life. And this system instills and inferiority complex into the Black culture, leading use to feel that white is right and that which is Black is wrong. This is why it is known as the greatest lie ever told. We must recreate our way of life spiritual system into one that represents the thoughts of

the Black woman and man. And this new system will bring fourth understanding of self and why God created mankind and what our purpose in life is.

Throughout history the Catholic Church waged war on all other religions. They tortured the Magicians, Priest, Witches and Warlocks whom practiced the religion of the Black race from Egypt. The Christian Pope's were key player in the start of the African Slave Trade, which lead to the deaths of millions of African people.

Today's churches or used as brain washing agencies for the ruling political party. Religion, Politics and Schools are said to be separate entities in the Western way of life. The political system rules all and affects all of these three systems. We must all realize that in life, all of these three areas are connected and have an affect on each other and your way of life. So they all must be brought into balance with each other. We can not say, do not kill in the churches then go out and wage political wars on other countries and kill innocent people. We can not say that churches or fine for society then turn a round and say that we can not have prayer in the schools.

Before the Christian Era the Egyptian People lived by the Maathian Creed which said your life should be ruled by Love, Truth, Peace, and Wisdom. This way of life system is contained in the 42 Laws of Maat.

The Christian religion took the Roman/Greeks hundreds of years to create. This religious system took the image of a Greek man by the name of Ptolemy and changed him into the Jesus Christ figure fore-which we know today. This religious system's first purpose was to deceive the Black Egyptian people but it's purpose now is to deceive all. Therefore the Christian Religion is manmade and not spiritually manifested. There exist no proof of the existence of the man known as Jesus Christ (Serapis). And the Biblical stories of Matthew, and John were created to give the elution of the existence of a man called Jesus the Christ.

When the Greek leader known as Alexander acquired rulership in Egypt, he demanded that the people worship him as a God. The Black people of Egypt refuse because they never worshipped human forms. They were in tune with nature and used their spiritual consciousness to guide them. This is the God-mind which is given to all, which links all of mankind to their spiritual consciousness, and the creator of all, God. After Alexander came the Greek leader named Ptolemy wanted to be worshipped as a God also. So he forced the Black Egyptian Priest to create the Jesus Christ story from the Ancient Egyptian stories of Isis and Osiris. The Greeks created various events around this Jesus Christ image and put the image in all the temples. The Black image of Osiris was removed from all temples. This image of Jesus the Christ was rejected by the Black Egyptians, so Ptolomy declared it illegal to practice the Egyptian way of life spiritual system and closed all Egyptian temples. All of the sacred Egyptian writing (scrolls) were removed from all temples. This was the start of the Roman Catholic Churches attempt to destroy The Black Egyptian Way of Life spiritual system.

Christianity's Attempt to Destroy the African Religious System

There was five original council meeting held by the Greek Ruling parties and the Roman Catholic Church leaders, that met for the purpose of making this Jesus Christ figure into a "God" and to eliminated the Ancient Black Egyptian spiritual system. The first meeting was held around 325 B.C. and the last of the five around 553 A.C. (B.C. - Before the Birth of Christ. A.C. - After the Death of Christ) Please note that the Bible has been rewritten many times throughout this long period of time, for one purpose, which is European or White rule over all whom which come under the Christian religion.

During the rulership of Constantine in Egypt, he stated that he would spread the Christian Jesus Christ stories throughout Europe, Africa and Asia. The Coptic Religious Community did not accept the Jesus Christ stories. So Constantine set out to destroy their religious worshipping system of the Divine Triad Of Isis (the Mother), Osiris (the Father) and Horus (the Son or child) which had been established by the Ancient Egyptian's.

Constantine with the aid of A Coptic Egyptian Priest named Sylvester started and spread the Christian religion out among the people. Sylvester was an

Egyptian Priest that gave in to the demands of the Roman/ Greek leaders, unlike other Egyptian priest whom fled or were put to death before they would give up their religious system. It took approximately 700 years for Roman/Greeks to get Christianity well spread throughout the region.

One of the Black Coptic Egyptian religious groups made a public statement that the Jesus Christ image was a falsely created image. And this same group started to fight against the Roman/Greeks Christian religious system. This group of Black Coptic Egyptian's were later to be known as Islam. (Coptic - means direct descendant of)

Later the Greek/Roman leaders held the Council of Nicene, in around 320 B.C. and 50 years later the council of Ephesus (430 B.C.). These two councils were held to erase the Ancient Egyptian definition of the Divine Triad (Isis (mother), Osiris (father), Horus (son)).

The Roman/Greek council inserted the Jesus Christ image into the Triad and he was to be now known as the Son of Osiris and Horus the son was excluded from the Triad, then later Osiris was replaced with the word father. And Isis was reduced to the image of the Virgin Mary. This was done to give the Jesus Christ image a spirit like nature and create a link between he and the Creator (God). Also it was done to give the Christ image a human form being born of the Virgin Mary and to reduce a womans purpose in life to domestic duties, erasing the spirituality that woman brings to this world. During the rulership of Theodosius I, and around 390 B.C. the council of Constantinople's was held in Constantinople's, Turkey. This council brought the false religion of Christianity in to full bloom by giving orders to destroy the Ancient Egyptian Temples. Destroyed along with these temples were the Ancient Egyptian writings (Religious Scrolls) for which were the only writings on the Earth that could be said to have been inspired by the Creator (God). It was know that the Creator (God) used our Black Egyptian Ancestors as messengers to bring fourth the God knowledge to mankind for the purpose of creating a spiritual and proper civilization for all of mankind.

At the Council of Chalcedon around (450 B.C.) the Greek/Roman leaders now stated that the false image of the Virgin Mary will be known as the mother of Jesus. And Jesus Christ will be viewed as both Son of God and God. At this time the man-made Christian religion had developed into the form for which we know it today. The creators of this new religion used it as a political tool to sway the people's mind-set in any direction they wanted to steer them (Brain Washing). During this time period the first Christian Roman Catholic Church was built called "The Church of the Blesses Wisdom". During the council of Constantinople II (550 A.C.) the Roman Emperor whom was also Pope of the Roman Catholic Church. Created the belief that the Pope was given the divine right by God (the Creator) to rule over the people. These type of council meetings are still being played out today but are hidden from the public.

We must always know that a Priest, or Pastor is not a requirement, but can only assist you in recognizing the God within you, which was put their by the Creator (God) so that each individual would know the Spiritual purpose of life. And from this she/he would acquire the ability to live a righteous life style. We must not let man made religious systems confuse us and alter our spiritual consciousness leaving us out of tune with the natural rhythms of Creation (God, Nature and the Universe). "If you can control how a person thinks you can be sure as to what actions she/he will take".

Origin of The Name Jesus

The Roman/Greek leaders after the invasion of Egypt created the image of "Serapis" in around 322 B.C..
Serapis was worshipped along with the Egyptian Goddess Isis, until approximately 430 B.C. when the Roman/Greek council changed the name Serapis into "Christ" and Isis was changed to Mary. This Christ image was also know as "Zeus" for the Greeks and "Jupiter" by the Romans and was still worshipped as a God In Roman/Greek Mythology. At the Roman/Greek Council of Lyons in 1245 A.C. the name "Jesus" was given to the Christ figure and this was done because one of the Black Coptic Egyptian religious groups had changed their Masia's name to "Muhammad". The Jesus image had previous names up until the time when the "J" was added to the Alphabet. The letter "J" was added to the Roman/Latin or English Alphabet in around the 1600 A.C.

The Muslim's (Islam) were one of the religious groups that fought against the Roman/Greeks Altering of the Black Egyptian Religious System. This Altering Created what is know as modern day Christianity.

The Ancient Black Egyptians practiced a way of life system that allowed them to be mentally in tune with the natural spiritual rhythm's of Creation or Cosmic Law, Called the Maathian Creed (Maat).

The Maathian Creed (Maat), Black Egyptian Yoga

The Maathian Creed Way Of Life System used a persons mental skills to take an individual up to his/her highest conscious state of being, which would give each person a highly enlightened spiritual state of being. This system was based on the acquiring of truthful knowledge and using this truthful knowledge in your everyday life experiences and actions. In this system a person's lower nature is suppressed while her/his higher nature is expressed in life. If a person bases their life on untruths (ignorant lower level thoughts and ideas) they will not be able to reach a calm state of being due to the disturbed uneasy mental state that is produced in the mind from the following of untruths. The Maathian Creed is expressed in the Ancient Egyptian Philosophy and Mythology. Egyptian Philosophy and Mythology should be viewed as tools to direct a person on how to live a righteous life. The morals in the Maathian Creed passage's are all that is required to be remembered and acted upon. These Philosophical and Mythological events should not be viewed as events that occurred some time in life but as moral guidance on how to live your life. During the time of the creation of the Black Egyptian Philosophies and Mythologies the world had in Egypt, the highest level of knowledge relating to the physical mental and spiritual components of life.

We must realize that civilizations knowledge level is not one directional moving first from the least knowledgeable level to higher knowledge levels as time passes on (Straight line). Knowledge is cyclic and is ruled by the Law of Rhythm that shows us that knowledge levels rise to a peak then fall to a lower level as time passes on and then repeats itself. This law explains why today's knowledge level is less than that of the time of the creation of the Maathian Creed, but some time in the future our knowledge level will be raised back to the Maathian Creeds high level and that time is the present Aquarius Age. One Great work of the Maathian Creed is "The Book of Coming Forth by Day and Night" ("The Egyptian book of the Dead"), which states that your spirit is sent to Earth (put in a human form) as part of the Creator's evolutionary process of purifying the soul. After the spirit or soul has reached its highest conscious level are purified state. The soul returns to the Creator (God). While practicing the Maathian Way of Life an individual must keep the company of persons of the same or higher conscious level so that she/he will raise their own conscious state of being and not lower it.

Historians have proved that the Ethiopian's (Nubian's, Egyptian's, Kemetian's) were the first of all men upon this planet and that all other men and races or an extension of the Black African Ethiopian people. Also that the Maathian Isis and Osiris stories were brought to Egypt by a colony of Ethiopians led by Osiris. India was another Ethiopian colony that practiced the Maathian Creed. The Maathian Creed was first written in Ethiopian Hieroglyphics. Hieroglyphics is a symbolic form of writing for which the writers were the only one's who understood the meaning of the symbols used in the hieroglyphics. Also historians show us that Egypt and India were invaded by various groups such and the Asiatics, Hiscos and Aryans, groups of people which later resulted in the lightening of the skin complexion and straightening of the hair of some of these people and a changing of some of their philosophies and way of life. It is also well know by historical scholars that the original books of the bible followed the Maathian Creed Laws and were later altered and some deleted by the Roman/Greek Christian Bishops for the purpose of deceiving the people for greed and power and not for the manifestation of Truth.

Understanding Spiritual and Human Existence

The Maathian Creed also states that all physical, mental and spiritual things in creation are a manifestation of the Creator (God). It goes on to state that the real and highest level of existence is that of the Spiritual state. Our earthly (physical) existence is just a mental manifestation coming fourth from our spiritual state of being. In other words our spirit is the only true level of existence and our earthly existence is just a tool used by our spirit to perform our earthly task of raising our conscious state to its highest level. Therefore our spirits self can be expressed as mental energy with a conscious purpose. If the human body dies before the spirit finishes it's task, then our spirit shall inter another body threw the process of birth. And use this body as a second tool to finish the earhly task. The spirit can also be defined as that life sustaining force of mental energy that is continuously passed from God to all things and which keeps all things existing as they do.

And The Creator (God) is the highest form of mental energy far surpassing the mental energy level of mankind. Due to the fact that we exist because the Creator's (God's) mental energy created us in the same form as his mental energy but yet at a lower level than that of the Creator. And this is why we have formed statements such as God created mankind in his own likeness, and we all have God with in us. This same mental energy that is emitted from the Creator is the same energy that God used to Create all in the Universe. For the fact that we are lower levels of God energy (mental energy), therefore being of God. If we learn all the truths of self, then we shall know God. Hence forth the statement "Know Thy Self".

In understanding that man is of the spirit and that his/her earthly existence is just a tool used by the spirit to carryout the purpose given to it by the creator. Then we must further state the fact that if mankind is of the spirit and is only using this earthly form for a Godly purpose. Then we must conclude, as the Maathian Creed states, that man's spirit is being reincarnated over a period of time. So when a person some time in the past died, his or her spirit at the time of birth entered another body in this present time to finished carrying out its spiritual purpose in the earthly form of a human being. And once a persons spirit has reached the highest mental conscious level she/he returns back to the source that brought it into being, the Creator (God). This is the true meaning of a person died and has gone to heaven. So in the dealth of a loved one we must not morn the loss but know that the person has moved back to its highest level of existence (Spirit form) and either will return back to Earth in another human body or be returned back to the Creator.

This modern way of life teaches us to think of children as a burden to the parent. The African way of life system taught us that a child was an asset to the family. We or all children of the Creator, do you think that we are burdens to the creator? No.

Our Mental Spiritual Conscious State of Being (42 Laws of Maat, Kabalion)

This leads us to wonder how can mankind raise them self's to the highest conscious level or highest mental state of being, as given to us, as our purpose of existing. When God (The Creator) let a spirit enter your body at birth each individual was given mental energy to be used to raise them selves to the highest conscious state of being. This mental energy shall be used to link your mind to your spiritual nature. Mental Energy can be broken down further into mental thoughts and mental thought patterns. For mental thought to be of the spiritual nature it must be true, because all that is of the Spirit is based on Truth and is of the Creator(God). This explains the meaning of the Devil or Satan which is merely the manifestation of wrongful or untrue mental thoughts. This leads use to express or purpose in life which is to gather up truths and to let or daily actions be guided by these truthful thoughts and to cast away negative or untrue thoughts. Now each person's actions can be guided by his/her higher spiritual nature. When your mind is in tune with your spirit your path to righteousness is straight and narrow. With this we must realize that mankind is of an earthly nature and is imperfect and will always manifest untruths in her or his life and must realize that the purpose of life is to push aside the untruthful things in life and follow the truthful things in life. This will form a pattern of truthful thoughts and actions. After many reincarnations each person will perfect this task of truthful mental thought and shall return to their spiritual existence with the Creator (God). Reincarnation is a state of being reborn again and again unto this Earth until a person has reached a certain degree of Spiritual Purity of their Physical Mental and Spiritual self. Once this is achieved the spirit returns to the Creator. Now we are back to the true meaning of returning to heaven (God). In this we must conclude that each woman or man at birth has the mental God given ability to decipher right from wrong and merely needs to follow and develop his or her truthful thoughts. Also we must note that no man requires another man to create for him what is truthful, for each person has that God (Creator) given ability. The man in the jungle that has no spiritual books has been given the ability to reach his/her highest spiritual state of being through her/his ability to decipher and act upon his/her truthful mental thoughts. But, a man can receive spiritual guidance from another man be she/he a priest, rich man, poor man, average person. The only requirement of the other man is that she/he be of equal or of a higher mental conscious state, so that she/he can aid the person in moving to a higher mental conscious state. The learning of truths and basing your actions on this knowledge is the learning of God knowledge which will intorn raise the conscious mind to its highest spiritual levels.

This leads us to the Maathian Creeds statement of "When the student is ready the teacher will appear". One of the meanings of this statement is that by the Laws of the Creator If any man seeks to follow his truthful (spiritual) nature he will be sent guidance in the form of a man whom which is of an equal or higher conscious state to further enlighten the person of the ways of truth and no man shall stop this process, for man is of a far lesser mental energy state than that of the Creator and must follow the laws of the Creator (God). Also dreams, thoughts, and energies (mental physical and spiritual) can be sent to the seeker.

The Creator's Mental Spiritual Energy is also described as Cosmic Consciousness which is to be understood as the highest level of mental spiritual energy in the universe that rules all other energy's in the universe and all other energies or derived from this first energy. We must note that the Creator made all in creation by way of Mental Spiritual Energy therefore all is of this energy. Giving meaning to the term "God is in all things", and "All thing in the universe or connected". If all things or connected then changing one thing must have an effect on another thing and the whole entire universe. This bring us to the meaning of, what you do comes back to you, and every cause has an effect. Each man or woman's mental thoughts and actions affect us all and it effects the entire universe.

The Black Egyptian Yoga system practices Meditative Prayer (self induced mental thought control) to aid a person in the manifestation of truth and the following of truth. The meditation practices will stop the production of untruths (wrongful thoughts) in the mind and will produce a proper mental spiritual mind set. This Yoga system taught the student to keep his mental state calm so that a person could think at their best. Also one of the Ancient Maathian Creed practices was to meditate (pray) to your ancestor's and ask them to aid and guide you in life, for they exist in the highest plane of existence the Spirit World and can aid you in life.

If a person tries to think when his mental state is at the extremes; sad, upset, happy, stressed out, then the persons mental processing is not at its best. A persons mind must be calm (balanced) for that person to utilize her/his mental capabilities at their highest level. Also you must not feed your mind untruths in the form of gossip, sex, violence, hearsay, lies, TV and Radio (Social Brain washing). These types of brain food will only produce bad thought processing in the brain. Remember that you will find some of the same or similar teachings in the Dogon, Hindu, Islamic, Buddhist, Zulu, Druids and other religious teachings for they all were derived from the Ancient Black Egyptian Maathian Creed teachings. Once a person has learned taught her/him self how to think properly and follow these thoughts in their daily actions, the person's life force energies shall be raised leading to higher physical, mental and spiritual state of being and awareness. One must also know that one's thoughts must first be from the heart then manifested in the mind. All thoughts and action must first originate out of Love because the heart keeps mankind truthful and passionate to all within nature and the universe.

The 42 Law's of Maat are righteous laws for developing truthful thoughts and actions that will lead a person to the obtainment of a higher conscious state of being. The practicing of Maat will calm and balance a persons mind and through the practice of meditation a person can reach a higher level of awareness of self and life. Please note that these 42 Laws are similar to the Ten Commandments but there are more of them. These Laws were in existence before the Ten Commandments. The Greek/Roman invasion of Egypt and the Creation of Christianity converted these Laws from 42 to 10 in number. See list of Laws below.

"42 laws of MAAT" (42 Rules of Righteousness)

1) I have not done unjust things
2) I have not done violence to anyone
3) I have not done violence to anything
4) I have not committed theft
5) I have not murdered anyone
6) I have not defrauded offerings
7) I have not acted deceitfully
8) I have not robbed the things that belong to the Creator
9) I have not told lies
10) I have not snatched away food
11) I have not spoke evil words
12) I have not attacked anyone
13) I have not slaughtered the cattle set aside for the Creator
14) I have not had deceitful thoughts
15) I have not done bad things to the Earth(soil) or that which grows from it
16) I have not been an ease dropper
17) I have not spoken against anyone
18) I have not become angry without cause
19) I have not committed adultery
20) I have not committed any sin against my own purity or the purity of others
21) I have not caused terror
22) I have not done that which is hateful
23) I have not been a person of anger
24) I have not acted against the ways of right and wrong
25) I have not stirred up strife
26) I have not caused any to weep
27) I have not lusted or committed fornication nor have I committed homosexual acts
28) I have not abused myself
29) I have not abused anyone or caused grief for anyone
30) I have not been overbearing on another
31) I have not judged hastily
32) I have not transgressed or angered God
33) I have not multiplied my speech over much
34) I have not done harm or Evil
35) I have not worked treason or curses on the king
36) I have never done bad things to the waters of the Earth
37) I have not spoken scornfully

38) I have not cursed the God
39) I have not acted with arrogance
40) I have not been overwhelmingly proud or boastful (ego tripping)
41) I have not increased my wealth except with things that or justly my own
42) I have never slighted the Creator

After a student has learned to master the 42 Laws of Maat and practice it in her/his every day actions. She/he can move to a higher level known as the Kabalion's Seven Hermetic Laws. These Laws govern and explains all things; physical, mental and spiritual energies in the Universe. These laws were said to have been written by the Black Ancient Egyptian Priest known as Hermes (Djehuti). Hermes is said to have reached the highest level in the Priest-hood of any man on Earth. Hermes also brought Astrology and Alchemy to mankind. George Washington Carver, a Black Scientist and Researcher, was the only know modern day Alchemist in America. This researcher never allowed books in the area were he was researching. How did he obtain so much knowledge? Yes, he meditated (prayed) to the Creator for the knowledge that he received.

Later this same Black Egyptian Priest (Hermes) was inserted into the Roman/Greek mythology as so many others were, and whose stories may have been altered by the Roman/Greeks for what ever purpose that they saw fit.

Kabala's Seven Hermetic Laws:

1.) The Laws of Mentalism
2.) The Laws of Correspondence
3.) The Laws of Vibration
4.) The Laws of Polarity(opposites)
5.) The Laws of Rhythm
6.) The Laws of Cause and Effect
7.) The Laws of Gender

The Laws of Mentalism
States that all is mind, meaning that all exist in the universal mind or from the God mind comes all.
Example: The Creators mind energy created all things in the Universe.

The Laws of Correspondence
Relates to the various planes of being, in life; As above so below, As in the macro as in the micro. (you or a duplicate of the universe, back to the term "Know They Self". When you understand self you will understand all in the Universe).
Example: The same Laws that apply to earthly things apply to all things in the Universe. The Creator is the Highest Level of Mind Energy and each person is a lower manifestation of this same type of mind energy.

Example: When you observe and atom you see electrons moving in various orbits around the nucleus of the atom, in the same way that the planets revolve around the Sun. The electrons and the planets or held in orbit around the nucleus and sun do to the electromagnetic energy (Life force energy) given off by the Nucleus and the Sun.

The Laws of Vibration
States that every thing is in motion (vibrates). Every thing physical, mental, and spiritual results from varying rates of vibrational energies.
Example: Every thing in the universe is composed of energy. This energy manifest itself into all the various things in the universe by transforming into various vibratory energy levels which intern creates all the things in the Universe. Therefore if all things are composed of some vibratory energy level then all things must vibrate and must be in motion.

The Laws of Polarity (opposites)
States that every thing is dual, has two poles.
Example: yen yang, good bad, right wrong, Woman Man, Masculine Feminine, Sun (positive) Earth (Negative), life Death, light darkness, East West
The law of polarity is continually working in our lives and this is why we have our highs and lows in life.
We can overcome the Law of Polarity by focusing in on the good in life and not the bad and search for the reasoning as to why a so called negative act or thing occurred.

The Laws of Rhythm
All things in life rise and fall
Example: Day always rhythmically flows into night. So does the seasons rhythmically change from one to another and then repeats. Your heart beat. The waves in the ocean. The Zodiacal Cycles of Time.
The Ancient Egyptian man had reached a very high level of understanding of self and his surrounding, after this age the world's knowledge level slowly declined but now the present Aquarian age energies will bring back that former high level of knowledge.

The Laws of Cause and Effect
Everything happens according to law, nothing just happens. No such thing as Luck.
Example: All things manifest due to some cause. If you do bad things bad things will come to you. So be sure that your actions are good so that good things will come to you. You are the cause of every thing that happens to you good or bad. Due to this law, you have total control of your life. I don't feel that God forgives you of your negative deeds because you created the negative cause and must suffer the negative effect in order to learn and grow to mental, physical and spiritual maturity. This law is evident in reincarnation. Some people start their lives off in bad conditions due to bad karma that they caused in a

past life and they must suffer the negative effects in the next life. Love is the performance of good actions (or causes) that bring forth good effects. So never argue with a negative are bad person because due to the Law of Cause and Effect, the harm that he or she commits shall eventually come back to them.

The Laws of Gender
This Law states that all things in creation have a masculine and feminine principle.
Example: All things in the universe have a masculine and a feminine state of being. Humans: Man brings the mental physical and woman the mental spiritual aspects to life.

Plants, animals etc. all have the law of gender expressed in their creation. Always remember that when dealing with the law of gender the two halves come to gather to make the whole. Examples: Man and woman unite to create the child. Man and woman unite in lasting partnerships in order to discover and understand their opposite nature (masculine or feminine) creating a well rounded and highly conscious being in each person.

We must realize that in creation there exist the Law of polarity that states: good and evil, right and wrong, shall always exist and is part of creation. So mankind will always encounter evil or bad things in life but a person must keep his mind-heart in balance and not let these things sway his/her positive mental thought processing.

Mankind's Seven Laws of Life (Written by the author)

1.) Keep the bodies energies Balanced at all time
2.) Keep your thoughts balanced and focused on the betterment of all in the Universe
3.) Keep your self in tune with the Cycles and Rhythms of the Universe
4.) Always remember that God (the Creator) is in every thing and is the controller of all things in the universe.
5.) Know your lineage (past history or ancestry) so that you shall know the future and what to due in the present time.
6.) Always follow truth and build upon your storehouse of truths
7.) Humans have a physical (animal or lower nature) and a Spiritual (righteous or highest nature). Spiritual existence is the highest level of existence and Physical existence is the lowest level of existence.

People who live their life's based on truth (the Laws of Maat) will no longer be concerned or attached to physical things of this Earth such as possessions, corrupt social and religious systems, the obtainment of money and power. These things only produce confusion and unrest in the mind. Once you start to live a life based on truth (Maat) then your mind will move toward a calm state which will enable you to rise to a higher mental and spiritual consciousness state of being. This new state of being will bring peace of mind and eternal happiness to the followers of Maat(Truth). The highest level of this new state is sometimes referred to as; raising the Kundalini (Serpentine Fire), the raising of your energies through the seven Chakra's of the Human body, or the seeing through the Third-Eye(spiritual self). Your Third-Eye is there to see things that your two physical eye's can not see, that which is of the mind and spirit. This is also the same as when God (The Creator) sends mental energy to a person in an attempt to raise the persons conscious state of being and awareness. This state of being is the ultimate goal of the Egyptian Yoga System. Which is to link mankind back to his spirit-self so that everyone's actions shall be guided by the Creator. The spirit-self is always at one with the Creator but is not the Creator nor does the spirit-self have power over the Creator (primary source of all things). The more a person strays from being mentally linked to her/his spirit-self the more he/she shall suffer from physical, mental and spiritual unease. Leading to a poor physical body condition, poor mental thoughts and no spiritual essence (guidance). The spiritual energies or the highest order of energy and if this energy is not present then all lower energies (mental and physical) shall decrease. Like wise if you develop your physical and mental energies then your spiritual energies shall be moved to a higher state.

This leads us to the fact that true reality is not in our physical existence but is in our spiritual existence and our mental state shall link the physical existence to the spiritual self. The body must use the mind to gain control over the physical senses so that it can move to a higher spiritual existence and awareness. When a person has formed a link between body, mind and spirit she/he may experience a feeling of Joy (similar to the shouting of a person in church), may become physic or may be fearful or confused but with the aid of a teacher the person will realize that they are starting to form a link with their real self (spirit-self). The person will learn, through meditative practices, that they have control of this spiritual state of being and may inter in or out of this state when ever they chose.

God created your spirit (god mind in everyone) and the spirit gathered up the elements and created the body so that it may prove that it is worthy of living in the spirit form. Once a person's spirit is worthy the cycle of reincarnations stops and the spirit returns to the maker (The Creator, God).
In the African way of life system, people who were on a high spiritual level were called Goddesses and Gods. This is comparable to the way some say that if you follow Christ you are a Christian.

Proof of the Existence of the Creator (God)

Modern science has proved that when they look into a substance they see smaller particles called protons neutrons, and even smaller particles, but as they look further into substances all they see is space (dark matter). And this substance is made mostly of this space (dark matter). In the Maathian Creed this space (dark matter) is defined as the God Energy that hold all thing together in their various forms in the universe. This energy is also referred to as Supreme Mind Energy which is energy with a mental purpose, being that of the Creator. This is more proof of the statements; God is in you and in everything, and all things or linked by the God Energy within them. When energy vibrates at high speeds it appears as light, when at low speeds it appears as matter. A good example of fast vibrating energy or the rays of the sun which penetrate the bodies of all things on this planet (humans, rocks , plants etc.). God Energy (Supreme Mind Energy), Life Force Energy or Spiritual Energy) penetrates into all bodies upon this planet in the same way that the sun's energy does. This is proof that the Creator (God) is the source of all things; our physical bodies, our mental thoughts and our spirit. So we are all manifestations of the Supreme Being but at a lower energy state. Each man/woman must "Know Thyself" fore then she/he shall know God because God is within every person and thing. Man must never try to match his/her intellect with that of the Creator (God) cause the creator is of a much higher Mental Energy state than that of mankind.

We may address the Creator using the name God, but we all know that the Creator has no name. And the Creator has no sex so don't call the Creator the Father, the Creator is the creator of all things the highest order of existence that can be perceived by man-kind. The living child is given to this world as a product of the Mother and Father. And the Creator is the mother and the father of all living things so if you call the Creator Father and not "Father/Mother" you or leaving out the Feminine part of creation, (see section on the Law of polarity (opposites).

Bodily Energies

Our bodily energies should be harnessed in the body and built up to their highest state because these bodily energies are used to fight off disease, heal the body and hold it in good health. Also it keeps the mind focused on positive righteous thoughts which raises your spiritual consciousness. When we loose our energies from worry, sexual intercourse, and negative thoughts such as greed, we bring forth unrest or disharmony in our energy systems of the body causing; disease, shortened life span, negative thoughts, mental stress, and a lowering of spiritual awareness. Fear causes the bodies electromagnetic energy level to be lowered which in turn lowers your energy level, conscious state of being and righteous path in life.

When we consume meat into the body it blocks the body from receiving the Life Force and Aquarius Age Energies from the Sun and Aquarius Constellation. (See Astrology Section for more info.) Meat also makes it hard for the Mind to concentrate and causes the body to loose energy that could be used for physical, mental and physic powers. Along with meat; drugs (over the counter and illegal), Alcohol, processed foods, unclean water, polluted air all cause a decrease in the bodies abilities. The cleaner the bodily systems are the easier the body can receive, retain and decode the light frequencies of positive energy. Melanin and clean water in the skin aids the body in receiving, storing up and processing the higher frequencies of Universal Energy from the Sun.

Chakra Energies

There are seven mental states of awareness, called the Seven Internal Chakra Energies (The Seven Seals, The Seven Breaths, the Seven Circles), that can be achieved. There are also 5 more Exterior Chakra Centers, giving way to a total of 12 Chakra Centers. The various state of mental awareness can be achieved through proper diet, good breathing techniques, meditative prayer, righteous thoughts and actions (42 Laws of Maat). "Note: It has been said that the brain's melanin content increases the more a person practices the Laws of Maat." One must have the proper knowledge and a relaxed or calm physical and mental state to raise his/her energies up to the Seventh Chakra (Third Eye, Raised Kundalini, Serpentine Fire communicate at your spirit level).

A person can have a Master Teacher give them instructions on how to raise their energies to the highest level. The Egyptian Caduceus, same symbol used by medical groups, is a symbol of the raising of ones energies to the seventh level. These energies are the physical energies of the human body. When these energies are out of balance in the body a person is more concerned with the negative or Un-Godly things in life. Endocrine System (glands) is the medical name for this group of Chakra energy centers.

But when these energies or balanced and moved up to the Seventh Chakra Level the person has learned to focus on positive things or Godly things (Truths) and now the person has linked her/his self with their Spirit-Self, where true existence and reality lies. The true meaning of marriage is in the Law of duality. A man and a woman's (plus and minus) energies become balance when they unite as one. This brings a balanced energy state where-bye the two can raise their energy levels and in turn raise their conscious awareness to the highest physical, mental and spiritual levels. At this seventh energy level a person is at their highest conscious state and can receive all the truths in the Universe. These energy centers relate to physical parts of the body which are controlled by the mind's positive electromagnetic thought vibrations: Base of the spine (Prostate Gland), Sexual organs (Gonad Glands), Navel region (Adrenal Glands, Solar plexus near the heart (Thymus Gland), Throat (Thyroid Gland), Brain (Pituitary and Pineal Glands). If you have a good memory there is a good chance you have a good functioning pineal gland. These glands work together in the physical storing up of electromagnetic energy and then mentally projecting this electromagnetic vibration out into the spiritual real of life, creating a communication link between the mental and spiritual self. Hence the need to purify and cleans the body and mind so that the body will take on it's proper energy flows and levels. One begins their building of energies in the Prostate and Gonad Glands of the sex organs. If one losses to much of these glands fluids (sexual intercourse, Masturbation, polluted body systems) one's energy levels (physical, metal and spiritual) will decrease along with his/her bodily functions. But if a person retains these fluids her/his energy level will increase, all bodily functions will increase and this energy can be used to raise the conscious level of the individual. (Note: a total absents of sex is not required and is similar to having to much sex, so a balance must be achieved for a person to achieve proper energy levels in the body.) The glandular system of the body has two functions one mental-physical and one mental-spiritual. When the energy level reaches the seventh Chakra (Pineal Gland) a person transforms from a mental-physical being and moves to a higher mental-spiritual state of being. In the human body the physical function of the glands are to secrete fluids throughout the body. But when your Chakra's are activated by the brains spiritual electro-magnetic thought activity these same glands produce a different type of fluid which is circulated from the prostate gland up through the spine to the other related glands and finally to the Pituitary and Pineal Gland. This process of the fluid moving from gland to gland and finally to the pituitary and pineal gland is what is know as the Serpentine Fire, Third-Eye vision, raising of the Kundalini or the moving of ones spiritual energies through the bodies seven Chakra points. Once the fluid or Chakra energy has reached the seventh Chakra (Pineal gland) the individual will become totally aware of their spiritual self (all Truths) and no longer be ruled by the ways of the material (physical world).

The Pineal Gland is the Seventh Chakra point and this gland is related to a person's ability to remember things. This is the same gland that produces Melanin in a Black person's skin, organs and body. The ability to remember is also related to the amounts of melanin in the brain cells. The more melanin (clean and un-polluted) the better the memory of the person.

The Spiritual function of the glands are very active in babies but the glands activity decrease as the child gets older. This decrease in activity is mainly due to a poor diet, poor mental teaching and polluted air. These glands also work in the immune system processes. The Thymus gland is one of the Chakra energy centers that assist a person in connecting to their higher self (spirit-self). This is why children are more spiritually connected to the God-Mind (spirit-self) within them than adults, also the fact that their minds have not been polluted with negative thoughts (Un-Truths) and have not been programmed to think a certain ways. Woman have a more well developed Chakra energy level (and memory ability) than men, due to the fact that their glands function better than men's. This makes the woman more in-touch with her spiritual self (more psychic) than men. And this is why you will find more women stating that they dreamed something and it came true. Or that they just know a certain something intuitively. Also this is why in the beginning of Egyptian culture The Woman Preceded the man in all rituals, on artifacts, in ceremonies ect… later on in time this system was reversed. The act of creation in humans is controlled by the women. The child is created in the mother's womb only when a woman allows a man to mate with her. And then after months of carrying the child the mother gives birth, fore she had total control of this act of creation.

The Adam and Eve story of the Bible is a depiction of the passing of energies from the Pituitary(Feminine) to the Pineal(Masculine) Gland which result in the enlightenment of the individual. The spiritual circuit is now completed (the (+) ("Electric", "Man") linked to the (-) "Magnetic", "Woman") equals energy. Man must learn about his feminine side and woman must learn about her masculine side.

All energies have an associated vibratory rate. The vibratory rate of the Chakra Energies or much higher than that of physical energies. Chakra energies are of the spiritual realm. The seven Chakra's control all energy levels in the body.

We must always remember that energies can be transformed by way of the thought process. What you concentrate on (think about each day), meditate and pray for is what you will become or manifest into this world and this is the "Law of Cause and Effect". So we should keep our minds in-tune with positive thought energies so that positive energies and events will occur in our lives. Mental energy (thought) by way of our spiritual powers can be transformed into physical things (physical energies).

In the beginning man had 12 DNA Chromosome Strands but to day we only have 2 DNA Strands. These 12 Strands gave man a number of abilities, such as physic ability, but we have lost these abilities. We had 12 DNA strands one for each sign of the Zodiac. The 10 lost Strands Equate to a loss of approximately 90 percent of our God given powers. These Chromosome strands affect you physically, mentally and spiritually and this is why we only use a small part of our brain functions in our daily activities. The present day Aquarius Age energies are being amplified by the Sun and are brought to your body (skin) in the form of Sunlight (life force energy). The melanin in your body is starting to decode these energies and is recreating the 10 lost DNA Chromosome Strains in the body. Also today's children or being born with more chromosomes, than the children before them. The way to gain back your 10 lost DNA Strands is to purify (cleanse) the body and the mind (mental thoughts) so that this new Aquarius Age energy can be processed by the human body. Correct mental thought processes can be obtained through the learning and understanding of the "Laws of Maat and the Law's of the Kabala". (The Kabala represents melanin in African rituals, ceremonies and writing's).

The Black African Man was originally a 12 DNA Chromosome Stranded being who at one point in time felt that he was equal to or greater than the Creator(God). So the Creator took away 10 of the Black man's DNA strands as punishment. Now after suffering the cause and effect of his negative actions, Karma, the time has come for the Black man to regain his 10 lost strands back from the Creator.

The Black person's body must absorb a lot of Sun Energy in order for it to speed up the process of recreating the 10 DNA Chromosomes Strains in the body. The more melanin (skin) exposed to the Sun's rays the more sun energy received and stored up in the body to be used in this regenerative process. A person will know if he or she is starting to pull in enough Sun Energy because they will start to see the Energy field "Aura" that radiate from the human body in all people. Also the Sun's energy is embedded in the air molecules, so do your breathing exercises.

We must realize that Mother Earth has the same Chakra Energy Centers as the human body. Man's wrongful deeds created a shift in the Earth's Chakra's from its normal energy levels. Now Mother Earth (Mother Nature) will force it's self back to its correct electromagnetic state. This is part of the reason why we or having and will have various changes in the weather patters, climates, storms, earthquakes, Volcano's eruptions floods ect…

Spirit-Self, God-Mind

We all have instances when our mind tells us to do things and we don't, then later on we say "I wish I would have done what my mind told me to do". This little voice in your head, subconscious thought, is the body's Spirit Self communicating with the mental self. If the mind is free of fear, hatred, Greed, envy, over inflated ego and other negative thought energies then the spirit self can easily link and communicate to the mental self. Or in other words we need to be made conscious of our Spirit Self. This is a proper state of being that has been lost due to social mental programming that has confused our minds and led masses of people to waist their mental energies on negative thoughts which produce negative actions. Our spirit self exist in a higher realm or at a higher vibratory rate than the physical and mental self. The Spirit Self does not have time restrictions put on it. It exists in the present past and future and this is why the Spirit Self can guide and aid you in living your life to the fullest of its potential. Now once we start to focus on positive thoughts and start to listen and follow our Spirits-Self (God Mind), we will realize first that this is definitely our Spirit-Self talking to us and that if we start to follow it the spirit is never wrong. Its purpose is to guide you and keep you righteous.

I was going to mail a letter one day and my mind told me to take the long way to the store and that I would meet a woman. I had been asking God to send me some one whom which I could communicate this Black Egyptian way of life system to. So when my mind told me to take the long way I told my mind no I am taking the short way. So I left out the door and the next thing I know is that I had taken the long way as my mind had told me. After I mailed my letter I turned and saw a women carrying bags and asked her if she needed a ride home. She said yes and we spent approximately three hours at her home and I told her all about the Black Egyptian Way of Life System and she thought this information was great. My meditative prayer had come true and my spirit self had guided me to it. Another example of being linked to your spirits self is that a lot of people, the vast majority of these people being woman, will go to sleep and dream things that will come true some time in the future. This has been termed as psychic ability or clairvoyance but it is merely a person who is more connected to their spirit self than others. My mom dreamed things all the time and these things later came true. Her mom dreamed of things before they happened also. One way to increase your connection to your spirit self is through good physical health practices, which intern calms the body and mind and increases the ability of your spiritual organs to do work. Then you must ready the mind to link to your spirits self by thinking righteous thoughts and doing righteous acts, Then you should use meditative prayer to calm the mind and connect you to your spirit self. All truths can then be manifested to you. Example: I was eating a good vegetarian diet, fasting meditating and asking god to aid me in raising my conscious level. Then one day I hade a dream that I had an African wedding in my mother's back yard and the lady I married gave me her birth date. I could remember the dream as if it had really happened. Three months later I was in an Astrology class and I meet a woman who looks just like the lady I married in my dream. I was spellbound, so I ask her what her birth day was and it was the same as the lady in the dream had said her birthday was, June the sixth. This woman's astrology sign was Gemini a sign that goes well with my sign Leo.

I feel that God sent me this dream in my sleep through my spirit self to prove that when women or men connect and let their spirit self guide them they can know all and they will be utilizing the highest level of mans abilities. God created a spirit in all things and this is what connects all things to one another. So when you connect to your spirit-self you are connecting to all in the universe, which intern gives you access to knowledge of all things in the universe. We say that God is in all things and that we or a part of God (Creator). So we all should have a permanent connection to God (Creator). This connection is the Spirit-Self.

Another thing that we must note is that which science has proved. The physical body does not require sleep to replenish it's self. The Ancient masters stated that the body rejuvenates its Spirit Self when we or sleep. Or to put it another way we form a closer connection with Spirit during our sleeping hours. And this is why people dream things and they come true.

We all should be working to raise the physical and mental vibrations of our bodies threw proper diet and good positive metal thoughts and analyses. When a certain higher vibration is reached by the human body that person automatically is linked to her/his Spirit Self. When a person attempts and in return starts to raise her or his conscious level to a higher vibration or energy state this new level of vibration will pull others and things to you which or of the same vibration as yours or higher, these people and things will aid you in moving to even higher levels of mental and spiritual knowledge, as stated in African Spiritual

Writings, "When the Student is Ready The Teacher Will Appear". So don't worry help is always on the way if you are trying to follow the righteous path in life.

Astrology (Numerology)

Astrology is the study of the vibrational energy forces in the universe and how these vibrational energy forces affect that which is in the universe. Numerology is another name which means Astrology and is a mathematical approach to deciphering the various vibrational energies in the universe, (The law of Cause and Effect). In Astrology mathematics is used as a tool to decipher and understand the different frequencies of astral energies and how these energies effect and interact with each other to form and maintain the universe. Man being part of the universe receives and interacts with these energies. And the understanding of these energies or translated into a worded form in today's Astrology books, so that the average person can better understand these energies. Astrology was brought to the world by the African Priest named Hermes and should be called African Astrology. Their exist African artifacts, calculations charts and tools that prove mathematics were well established in Africa 26 thousand years ago. So the African must have started mathematics some time even further back in history.

Astrology and Occult Metaphysics go hand in hand. Occult means something that is hidden and Metaphysics means that which is above. So Occult Metaphysics is the study of the hidden energies that reside in the universe and or controlled by the Creator.

Many thousands of years ago the Black Egyptians studied the Celestial bodies (stars planets) in the northern, southern and central section of the sky and represented each section as a Circle divided into 12 smaller sections each representing a sign of the Zodiac. These three sections together were represented as three interlocking circles and these circles have been found in various places all over the Globe (another trinity). On the ceiling of the Pyramid's of Giza you will find various star structures and all twelve signs of the zodiac.

The African Dogon people of Mali possess a highly genius level of understanding of Astronomy (Astral bodies in the universe), and the physical composition of all things (matter), such as atoms, genetics, etc.

Below is a list composed of the different manifestations of the Life Force Energy (God Mind Energy). All energy's of any type comes first from The Creator's "God Mind Energy" and then later is broken down into the various different types of energies.

God Mind Energy = Life Force Energy = Creators Energy = Frequency = Energy = Vibrational Energy = Electric Energy = Electromagnetic = Magnetic

Energy = Mind Energy = Physical Energy = Healing Energy = Spiritual Energy ect...

Please remember that all in the universe is made of energy at difference vibrational frequencies. All electrical energy sources have an associated frequency. (Example: your outlets in your home where you plug your appliances in is a 120Volt energy source with a frequency of 60Hz.) Your body has electrical energy passing throughout it by way of your nervous system, and your body gives off an associated frequency (Aura) which is generated by the energy from the body. All bodies (Man planets, thoughts ect...) and things in the universe have an electrical energy state and an associated frequency.

A radio station broadcast a particular radio show to your radio at a particular frequency and you tune your radio to that frequency (Example 105FM) and now you receive what information that is being broadcasted to your radio from that Broadcasting Station. This is the same way in which all things in the universe interact with each other. In astrology a particular planet or body in the universe gives off a certain frequency which is broadcasted through space to Earth and then received by your body. When you were born the Sun was in one of the various Zodiac Signs (Cancer, Leo, Aries ect...). If the day was July the 15th, the Sun was broadcasting the energy frequency of "Cancer", which gives the person the Astrological Sun Sign of Cancer. This frequency of energy interred your body and created part of you mental personality and the other bodies in the universe also were broadcasting different frequencies of energy that interred your body and played a part in developing your total personality. Such as if the moon was broadcasting the Leo energy frequency on July the 15th at 5:00pm, then your Moon sign would be Leo. The various personality traits mentioned in astrology books are just a worded explanation of the various frequencies of energy given off by the associated planets or bodies in the universe. (See section on Kabala's Laws of Correspondence) This interaction between bodies (planets and humans) in the universe is the Creators (Gods) way of providing our planet with all the various personality types required to create a proper and righteous society. Samples of various personality types can be seen below:

Zodiac Sign	Personality Type	
Libra	Judges, Lawyers	
Pisces	Priestess, Mystic	
Leo	President, Leader	
Aquarius	Scientist, Humanitarian	
Aries	Pioneer, Warrior, Leaders	Ect...

(Note: The Sun (hot) is the youngest of the Astral bodies in the universe and the Moon (cold) is the oldest. Due to the fact or law that all things in the universe gravitate from a state of hot to a state of cold, as the body losses heat energy.)

Sunlight makes plants grow and a similar process is carried on in the human body. Melanin covers each cell of the body. When the sunlight frequencies are absorbed by your skin. These sun frequencies or amplified by Melanin and water in your skin and past on to the cells of the body and activates various DNA chains in the cell of the body. In this same way astrological and Zero-point energies affect the human body and mind. Also this is how Aquarius age and other age energies or pasted on to the human body. Sunlight transmits data to the human being in a similar way as the modern day Fiber-Optic (light) Systems transmit light encoded data, and Satellite, Phone and radio systems transmit frequency encoded data. (See section on The Laws of Correspondence)

We could create the perfected society by motivating Pisces people to take on life interest in Mysticism and Religion, Libra's life interest in Justice, Leo's in Authority positions, Aquarius's in the Sciences ect.... If you take on these particular interest then you are involved in the area of life that God put you here to be involved in. Therefore you shall excel much faster than others and be much happier in life, fore you have aligned your thought processing energies to the area that your mind works best.

In Ancient African Tradition people were married in accordance to their astrological sign compatibility. Also in ancient times their existed African groups that were named after the various zodiac signs and all the members of that group were of the same zodiac sign. This method of living would propel each member in a tribe to her/his highest level of understanding when it comes to his/her personality type (Know Thy Self). Astrology is the Creator's (God's) recipe for society and should be taken very seriously by all.

We must know that Astrology was first and then all the other subject matter such as Maathian Creed Laws, Kabalion's Laws and other Black Egyptian teaching sprang forth from the African Astrology teachings.

Astrology states that the moon emits a feminine energy. And this energy can be felt at its highest during a full Moon, which occurs once each month. A good example of African Astrology in our every day lives is the effect the Moon cycles have on humans. During the time of a Full Moon, we receive the maximum amount of energy from the moon. The Full Moon energy is felt by man and amplifies her/his emotional state. In astrology the moon rules the emotions. If you were to go to a police station and review their records it would show that they have more calls during a full moon than any other time. Emotional things such as arguments between family and friends are common during this period of time. So be sure to keep a positive loving emotional state during Full Moon Days, don't be negative because your negative emotions will be amplified even greater during Full Moon days. This is due to the fact that electrical currents in the body shift with the Moon's Zodiac Cycles.

We receive energy from each planet or body in or universe and each one has a part in developing our total personality. Each planet has cycles and therefore some energies or higher or lower at different times of the year. A person can use these cycles to determine when a certain type of energy is high and now they have a better chance at performing a certain task because the energy is there to aid them.

A good way to test if Astrology is based on truths is to read the Sun Sign personality description of family members and long time friends. You will find out that each person is a lot like their Sun Sign personality description and that members with the same sign or a lot alike and members of others signs or a lot different from each others. Also you will see many other relations that prove African Astrology is based on truth.

Four major areas of a person's African Astrology description are the Sun Sign, Rising or Ascendant Sign, Mid-Heaven or MC Sign, and Moon Sign. The Sun Sign is a description of the person's basic personality traits (70%). The Sun Sign has the most influence over a person because the Sun is a Star and not a Planet and a Star has greater powers than that of planetary energies. This is why the Sun is the ruling energy source in our world. The Rising Sign is how people view you as a person and is approximately 30% of your basic personality. The Mid Heaven or MC is your purpose in life. This is the job that the Creator(God) sent you hear to perform. The Moon Sign will show you what type of basic emotional traits a person posse's. The various personality traits given to a person can be used to match that person with a mate that is compatible with them. Also African Astrology will reveal a person's good and bad qualities.

African Astrology has various Zodiac Cycles contained within it, such as the Stellar, Lunar and Solar Calendars, that one should learn about. Another particular cycle is the Great Year Cycle (26,000 years) that states that the Earth spins Approximately 2,200 years in each Zodiac Sign. Which means that those particular attributes of the sign are heightened during that Age. Example: We or presently in the Aquarius Age which means that Truth Seeking (Spirituality), Science, and Humanitarianism will be at its highest point during this age. Which means that during this age mankind will learn all the Truths about religion, science and self. And that he/she shall perform more humanitarian acts than ever before. We just came out of the Pieces Age, which was the age of religion, and deception. And this is why we have had so many religions and religious wars since the fall of Egypt. There is an over lapping of energies at the end points of one age and the start of the next age and this is why some have predicted the fall of Christianity (Roman Catholic Rule) in the next 10 years. This is the end of the Pieces Age(religious deception) and beginning of Aquarius Age energies which bring forth Truth. Prior to the Pieces age was the Aries Age which is ruled by Mars which brings forth energies of Aggression, Conflict and new beginnings. And this is why in this period of time Egypt was being destroyed by internal chaos and repeated invasions and wars by other groups of people. And after the fall of Egypt, end of the Aries Age, the world lost its great mass of knowledge and had to start all over again. And this was the start of a new Astral life cycle upon this Earth which is now in the Aquarius stage of the cycle.

Also the Aquarius Age Energies are said to be the cause of the Million Man March in Washington and the Woman's Rights Movement, giving way to a resurgence of African thought in society, which includes putting the feminine essence (spirituality, love, beauty etc..) back into our society. If you have made a positive significant change in your life or life's path, this also is due to the new Aquarius Age Energies affecting your body and your actions in life. (One of the African symbols of the Aquarius Age is the Black Ethiopian King). These new Aquarius Age Energies are bringing higher level souls to this Earth in the children that or being born today, and today's children or very strong beings. Below is a chart of four different Ages and the time (years) that they occur in. Also a chart of the Planetary relation to the days of the week.

The Earth spins approximately 2,000 years in each African Zodiac sign!

Age	Date Aprox.	
Aquarius	2000 AD -- 4000 AD	("Present Time")
Pieces	0000 AD -- 2000 AD	
Aries	2100 BC -- 0000 AD	
Taurus	4000 BC -- 2000 BC	

Planet to Days Relation Chart

Monday	------	Moon
Tuesday	------	Mars
Wednesday	------	Mercury
Thursday	------	Jupiter
Friday	------	Venus
Saturday	-------	Saturn
Sunday	-------	Sun

The book of "Enox" that should be in the bible was taken out because it is all about Astrology The writers of the bible did not want the people to know about Astrology. But you can still find Astrology related information in the bible such as the 12 Tribes of Israel relates to the twelve Zodiac signs.

We are presently in the Aquarian Age. The Aquarian Age energies shall reach there maximum output to Earth during the mid-point of its 2,200 year cycle. Then it will slowly decrease and the next Age's energy will come into being on Earth. The Aquarian age energy has also been referred to as the Schumann Resonance Energy. (Example: A way to describe this Aquarian energy source is to take a small ball and roll it around the edge of a round table and at one

point on the table's edge, shine a flashlight. At one point in time the ball will roll into the area of the table were the beam of light is shining down on it. This is the same way that the Earth now has the Aquarian age energy shining down on it.)
Zero Point is a high energy state that has been referred to as a time when the Earth will stand still for a moment and then reverse its direction of rotation, due to a shift in the polarity of the Earth's North and South poles. Ancient Black cultures such as the Egyptian's, Dogon and Mayan's have recorded history of this event happening many years ago, and that the next occurrence of Zero Point will be on December 21, 2012 during the "The Winter Solstice". "The time when the Goddess will be awakened in us all". Some of the records state that the Sun began to set in the West and reversed its direction and back tracked across the sky and sat in the East. This event gave the people of that region 24 hours of sun light instead of 12. Other records speak of a longest night, that lasted 24 hours which would be what happened on the other side of the earth.

It has also been said that during this moment in time that the Earth stops rotating, and the Earth's magnetic field will also stop being emitted from the Earth, due to the lack of rotational energy to generate this field. This lack of a magnetic field on the Earth will allow the Earth to receive its largest amount of Aquarian Age energy, fore which all on Earth shall receive. And this energy will change (raise the vibrational rate of) all things physically, mentally and spiritually. At this time man shall receive, (If he ask), all the knowledge of self and live in a world based on truth (utopian society) and man shall have access to all truths.
(Utopian - a society with the ideal social, political and spiritual structured.) (This is the True meaning of the second coming of Christ in the Bible.) These new vibrational frequencies will usher in a new evolutionary period for all upon this Earth.

Universal Energies

The spinning of the different layers of the Earth in different directions produce and electromagnetic type of energy, which is projected out into the universe. And when the Earth is in its reverse phase it receives energy from the Sun and this energy spins the earth on its axis and rotates the layers of the Earth. The layers of the Earth or similar to the magnetic-coil configuration of a motor or generator, which inputs and outputs electric energy. In Astrology different frequencies of this electromagnetic type of energy is produced by all Astral bodies (planets, stars, humans) in the universe, and is necessary for the existence and connectivity of all things in the universe, from the Macro to the Micro. Fore it is this energy (cause and effect) that binds together all things in the universe.

Life to Death

The moving from the living state to the state of being dead is only a transformation from one Physical, Mental state to another Mental, Spiritual state of existence. The person or thing goes from one energy state to another energy state. All things are just different manifestations of Mental Energy, and the Creator is the highest form of Mental Energy, who controls all energies.

GOD "CREATOR"

God is the Universal energy or electromagnetic vibrational force that exist in all things and which keeps all things in motion or alive. The African Egyptian symbol for God is a circle with a dot in the middle. The meaning of the symbol is that God is the center or controlling mind of all things and she/he transfers his/her energy out to all things is the universe. Some of us question the existence of God (Creator). My answer to this question is for the fact that I exist, some higher order of being had to create me and all other things in the universe. Science has proven the existence of the creator when they look at any substance through a microscope they see molecules then atoms then protons neutrons and electrons and even smaller particles than these but the final thing that they can detect is the space between these particle for which is the God Energy that holds all thing together and in their place. (Example: like a magnet holding a pin.) And this is why we say God is in all things. This Universal God energy is sometimes referred to as the law of Attraction are the Law of Love. Love holds people together and in their proper state in nature but hate disrupts you and takes you out of balance with nature.

God (The Creator): = Righteousness = Truth = Love = Harmony = Peace

Aura

In the various sections above we have discussed the body and it's electric nature. The aura is the high frequency electromagnetic light energy that is given off of a body do to the body's electrical frequency. The body's frequency is directly related to the conscious level of the individual. Basically the body's energy gives off light in the same way that a light bulb's energy gives off light but at a much higher and different frequency. Aura's can be seen by the human eye if the person is in the proper state on being.

Example: At a time when I was fasting, meditating, having a proper diet, and reading spiritual books, and focusing my mind on spiritual things, I went to a health seminar and a very dark-skinned brother stood up and asked a question and the speaker said that he could see that the guy was of a higher consciousness because he could se the yellow aura that was encircling his head like a hallow. He then said that some of you out there will be able to see this aura but some of you will not. I turned and looked at the guy and I could see the yellow aura just above his head. Then I looked a round at all the other people and I knew that they could not see this Aura. I feel that I was in the proper receptive state to see the human aura and this is why I could see it and others did not. The bodies aura is said to change color in regards to the physical health of the individual also. This Aura has been used by healers to detect illness in the body. Women's Auras are larger that men's due to the more Spiritual nature of the woman.

Pyramids

There or many African Egyptian Pyramids all over this planet that were all constructed by our Ancient Black Ancestors. All of the Ancient Artifacts and pyramids found all over the world have Black peoples faces on them with thick lips and pug-like noses and woolly hair. Researchers have concluded from the gathering of measurements, astrological and various other types of data found in the pyramids that all the pyramids around the world originated from one source, The Black Egyptians. And everywhere that we see these African pyramids there was a temple of learning were the people of that area would go to learn the righteous teachings of the Creator (God). Modern day space exploration equipment has found and taken pictures of African pyramids and a Sphinx on the planet Mars and also they have found pyramids on the Moon. The Mars pyramids have been dated back to approximately 500,000 years ago. Before these modern day so called discoveries, the Ancient Zulu and Dogon people of Africa, had long since stated that there were pyramids on Mars and the Moon. The Amazon Jungle is the home of thousands of African pyramids. In the Amazon Jungles there is proof of irrigation and other systems required to maintain a large society that show that a massive civilization of millions of people once lived there. There also exist what is called the Blue Green Pyramids that exist underneath the Oceans and it is said that the crystals in these pyramids still function. Easter Island and regions in China, British Isles and Japan are other area's were African pyramids exist. A number of top Geologist and Archeologist have stated that the Sphinx is at least 20 to 30 thousand years old and Ancient Black Egyptian writing's state that the Sphinx and the three neighboring Great Pyramids of Giza date back to the beginnings of mankind's existence on this planet. The Sphinx which has a human head and a lions body represents the Leo Constellation of stars and the face is that of a woman representing the spiritual nature in the world. Other Specialist say that the pyramids are around 300,000 years old. Pyramid Mathematical calculations and measurements have revealed the exact length of the calendar year and the time it takes for the Sun to make one revolution in space, which is the time it takes the sun to travel threw all Twelve Star Constellations of the Zodiac known as the Great Year. The Great year is approximately 26,000 years which means that each Zodiac Star constellation has a length of approximately 2,200 years.

A lot of the still existing pyramids have been labeled as "Earth Mounds" this is incorrect! Over a long period of time (thousands of years) the wind has blown debris over the Step-Pyramids covering them with dirt and this is why they appear to look like an Earth Mound. The African Mound Builders were the creators of the pyramid known as Monks Mounds located next to the city of East

St. Louis, Illinois just off the Mississippi River. They built pyramids in the St. Louis Missouri area also. Artifacts have been found that give proof that the Mound Builders, The Indian's of North America, Cherokees, Hopi etc., were Black people. Also the Black people of Mexico known as the Omex build hundreds of still existing pyramids in Mexico. The Omex's of Mexico were Astrologist whom which carried on a vast study of Astronomy. The Omex's left large black stone statues with the faces of black men on them which prove who these people were.

One of the most well known historical institutes have found and destroyed many African Artifacts that were found in and around the pyramids and in the Grand Canyon Caves in America and have others stored a way out of the public eye.

The African Mound Builders lived in circular pyramids constructed dwelling (cone Shaped) called Tee-Pee's. The Mound Builders the Black African Egyptians and the Omex people of Mexico are all African Descendants. Historic writing's state that around 1500 BC there was a catastrophe (Earthquake and Flood) which separated The America's (North and South) from Africa which at one time was one large land mass, and this is the story of the parting of the sea's and the great flood in the Bible. Also their have been seven great floods during man's existence on the Earth. "I predict that their will be a Great Flood within the next 12 years which will flood the Mississippi Valley Area, and cover the Monks-Mound Area. Later the waters will recede uncovering and revealing the actual granite pyramid underneath the mound. Also their will be a series of Earth Quacks that will rejoin the American and African Land Masses back together as they once were." A large number of burial sites and remains have been found in North America. At these sites the people buried their dead in the fetus position with their faces toward the North which is the same burial methods as the Ancient Egyptians. Researchers conclude that these remains are that of a people whom existed at lest 100,000 years ago and are of African Egyptian descent. It has been proved by science (study of the structure and chemical composition of rock and soil) that the geological make up of the soil in North and South America is the same as that in Africa, so the three regions had to have been one large land mass at one time. If you take South America and pull the land mass over to Africa and let Brazil connect to Nigeria you will see that they fit together like the pieces of a puzzle, giving physical proof that they were once connected as one large land mass. Along with the Pyramids various other structures that exist today were built by the Egyptians such as the Stonehenge (Egyptian Temple) located in the British Isles.

The Hieroglyphics in the Great Pyramids are eroding away and will be gone in approximately the next 100 years. This is due to the fact that the new Aquarius Age Energy will bring forth truth (true knowledge) to all, so their will be no need for the hieroglyphs to guide humanity.

The pyramids around the Globe were built by the Ancient Black Egyptian peoples led by the knowledge of the ancient priest. Each pyramid is located at a point on this Earth were the life force energy is being emitted back up out of the Earth at a higher level than that in other surrounding area's. This is the same life force energy that is being emitted by the Sun that keeps all things on this planet alive. The Sun forces this life force energy deep into the Earth and this energy is later re-emitted out of the Earth (The Earth & Sun energy cycle). And large amounts of these energies are being re-emitted from the Earth at the various pyramid sites. Each pyramid is located over an underground water source (battery). Each pyramid (energy point on the Earth) represents one of the Earth's Chakra Energy Centers and each pyramid carries an energy level relating to that particular Earth's Chakra Energy Level. These Earthly Chakra Energy Centers are a working energy grid that encircles the globe. (see section on Human Chakra centers and section on the Kabala's Law of Correspondence). Some of the pyramids on the Earth have been destroyed. The destruction of these pyramids has thrown the Earths Chakra Energies off (Energy system off). The Earth is now in a process of rebalancing the earth's energies and this process calls for the shifting of the Earth's tectonic plates (earthquakes) and odd weather systems (floods, tornadoes) as the Earth's environment rebalances itself. We must note that there is a need for negative energies (Physical, Mental and Spiritual) in the world. Negative energies bring forth change into positive and balanced energy states. The present day negative actions and things shall in the near future bring forth a positive and balanced state of being in the world, then the cycle (Great Year, (26,000 years)) will once again repeat itself.

The underground water source in the pyramids are used to store up the life force energy that is being re-emitted from the Earth, in the same way that you charge up a battery. Later this life force energy is pasted through the pyramid were it is amplified by crystals and sent up and out the top of the pyramid. Therefore the pyramid was engineered in a way that its structure would store-up, contain and amplify this life force energy. And our bodies store-up, contain and amplifies the life force energies contained in it. (See section on Chakra Energies) The human body stores up energy in the sex organ region of the body by way of physical and mental power. This energy is raised and amplified up through the body's (spinal-cord) and emitted through the Crown Chakra (pituitary and pineal glands) located in the brain out into the spiritual realm of existence (your spirit-self).

Due to a woman's physical make-up, construction of the sex organ region, a higher water content and different mental state of being a woman was designed by the Creator in a way that she can heighten her spiritual awareness or awaken her God Mind (spirit-self) faster and much easier than her male counterpart. (see section on The Maathian Creed (Maat), Black Egyptian Yoga). The pyramid was used to aid a person in putting her/his body back to the proper electromagnetic frequency or vibration and to aid the person in the act of raising their energies to the spiritual level which would return her/his body back to its original or proper state, "at one with nature(creation)".

The pyramid energies that or being emitted have a second function which is to form an energy grid around the Earth which will hold the Earth and everything in and on the Earth, at its proper energy state or frequency, "at one with nature (creation)". The priest designed the pyramids to hold the Earth's atmosphere at the proper vibration or energy state and the alteration and destruction of some of the pyramids around the globe has altered the Earth's balanced energy state and in return has altered man's physical and mental state of being disconnecting us from our spiritual self's hence, creating the society we live in today. We have to regain our proper state of being so that we can return to being a people at one with creation (the Creator).

Please note: That a pyramid is simular to a parabolic dish antenna (round antenna you see on peoples houses for cable T.V.) put face down on the ground so that the energy received from the Earth can be gathered up by the wide base of the pyramid and then amplified by a crystal in the center of the pyramid and transmitted up and out of the tope of the pyramid, in the same way that a parabolic dish antenna pulls in the satellite transmitted signals (various cable station channels) that are sent to your T. V. A Black persons body has this same function it pulls in and stores energy in the melanin of the skin and then amplifies and transmits this energy up through the Chakra energy centers and out the Pituitary and Pineal Glands to the Spiritual World to all that exist in the universe; physical, mental and spiritual. But one's body must be purified (clean) and one's mind must be righteous then a person can transmit and receive this Spiritual Energy (connect to her/his Spirit Self). This is why the Yoga sitting position resembles a pyramid, your legs and base of the spine represents the base of the pyramid and your Brain's Pituitary and Pineal Glands represents the crown of the pyramid (the top, cap-stone, crystal transmitter).

Ankh Symbol of Life

The Ankh was first found in Egypt. Some say that one of the oldest Black Egyptian Ankhs is stored a way in the Vatican. Most Ankhs are found attached to a power unit called the Djedi. The Ankh represents a balance between opposites, such as positive and negative. It is called the cross of life. It represents eternal life in all things. It has been said that the vibrational energy from the Ankh can be transmitted to any person or thing near the Ankh and that this energy will give that person the energy of life. The loop at the Top of the Ankh is said to be able to transmit and receive energy. Science has long since known that energy can be transmitted through Melanated skin. The more melanin ("a metal compound that can transmit, receive or store-up electrical energy") in the skin the more energy you can pass through the skin. The Ankh was used in

Ancient Egyptian times to transmit and receive energy to and from the body, by holding it in the hands of a person. The person's state of mind was the tuner that determined what kind of transmission and at what energy level. The staff that Moses carried in the Bible stories was a Djedi with an Ank attached to the top of the Djedi. This unit by way of mental thought control (mind over energy) pulled in life force or magnetic energy and redirected it to perform various task. Crystals were used in the construction of some of the Ankh's which gave the unit the ability to resonate it's energy at the same resonance frequency of the crystal.

Note : All things resonate at some energy level given to it by God the Creator of all energies in the universe" When these frequencies of energy combine with one another new substances, thoughts and things (Physical, Mental and Spiritual) are created. Example; when we add microwave energy to a cup of water in a microwave oven the water heats up and is transformed into stem.

Another meaning of the Ankh is that it represents the sex organs of man and woman "Creation". The top loop represent the woman birth canal and the staff the males penis and the cross-bar the Gonad Glands.

Black Man, The 1st and Only Man

Archeologist have proof that the first man known to exist on this Earth was the Black people known as the Pygmy. The decayed bodies of Ancient Pygmy people have been found in various places around the world some in America and some have been dated back to around 600,000 years ago. These people were the first Egyptians. Ancient Egyptian Artifacts (drawings) show the Egyptians of that time as having the same characteristics as that of the Pygmy. The oldest of African remains date back to approximately 750,000 years ago. And other descendants of the Pygmy people or the Black Ethiopians, Black Nubians, Black Aborigines, Mayas people of Mexico, Incas people of South America, Black Druids, Black Dogons, Black Zulu's American Indian's Cherokees, ect… All these groups shared the same African Phenotype (visible properties, bone structure and skin), African Genetics, African rituals, and Social practices (art, writings, architecture, tools ect…). We must remember that in ancient times, various glacial episodes have occurred in apox. 26,000 year intervals that forced some of the ancient people to move to different regions of the world were the climate was suitable for living. And this is one of the ways mankind has been spread out over the different regions of the world.

When we go back in time all we see are these Black group of people whom lived in warm Climates, Africa. Then later on man moved out from Africa to other parts of the world to semi-cold and cold climates, and today man exist in many different climates around the globe. The Creator put the first man in a

Warm Climate (Africa) so that the man would retain and have access to all of the essential elements for life. One of the main elements that man has retained due to staying in a warm climate is the Melanin content in his/her skin (body). A warm climate gives way to out door activities and less clothing so that the Sun's rays can be absorbed by the human body and in return produce more melanin (sun tan). The Creators gift of Melanin aids the Black man in raising his physical, mental and spiritual self to the highest levels, ("if only that man chooses to raise his or herself"). (See section titled "Melanin") It has been known by scholars that if a Black group of people moves from a warm climate to a cold climate this same group of black people a thousand to two thousand years later will now be termed as white people due to the lost of color (melanin) in their skin and body. This lack of melanin was caused by man not receiving adequate amounts of sun light energy to the skin and Body. A cold climate gives way to less out door activity and more clothing therefore man receives less sun energy to the body. Also the hair will go from curly and dark to straight and not so dark in color due to a lower content of melanin. The energy from the sun keeps the melanin producing glands (Pineal) active and functioning at full capacity. The lack of the sun energy decreases the functioning of the melanin producing gland so it becomes calcified and produces less Melanin and in return the body's physical mental and spiritual abilities are also lessened to some degree. This is the reason why I feel Racism against the Black African People exist all around the world.

Please note that if the Sun was to stop shinning down upon the Earth all living things would soon after die. The Sun's energy sustains all life upon this planet with out it we and all living thing will die, I thank the Creator (God) for giving the Sun's energy to the world. (The Laws of Correspondence - relates to the various planes of being in life, as above so below, as in the macro as in the micro). The magnetic pull of the Sun hold's all of the planets in our solar system in orbit around it and in return baths the planets with its sun energy.

Future

In the near future there will be many earthquacks, floods and other catastrophes that will occur around the world. I feel that the earthquacks and floods will be a direct result of the New World Order Wars that or taking place today. Science has proved that the debris from wars collects in the upper atmosphere and circles the globe creating a warming affect and a depletion of the ozone layer all over the Earth. This warming effect will cause glacial melt downs which will create flood conditions all over the globe and nature will bring forth great rains in an attempt to cleanse the air and upper atmosphere. Earthquacks will be generated due to the depletion of resources from the Earth (oil, coal, iron, ect...), the shock waves and it's vibrations which or being emitted into the Earth from the bomb blasting in the wars will trigger earthquacks. The melt-down of glaciers will create a need for the Earth to rebalance its land masses by shifting them to a different position until a balance is reached. Then a great shift of the

Earth's poles will occur in order to cleanse and rebalance the Earth and all within it. (See section in this book titled Astrology "Zero Point") But after the great shift of the poles of the Earth a new government based on Love for all man-kind will be put into place world-wide. And man will live in harmony, having peace on Earth, love for one another and no more fear. And only then will all of mankind be put back to their proper and balance mental, physical and spiritual state of being. The Mayan's predicted that a new Evolutionary Cycle for mankind will start on December, 21 in the year 2012. Various African Indian Chief's (Shauman, Priest) broke their code of silence and or telling the ruling forces of today that their ancestors predicted the down-fall of their rule in the near future (with in 10 years). Also they predicted that Idaho, Wyoming Washington, Nevada and California will all get flooded and or washed away.

Illuminati

A number of the high ranking political and religious leaders or part of the Illuminati. Also many of our large scale corporations or part of the Illuminati. It has member from all races. This is a group whose main purpose is to obtain power, world control and resources by any means. They rule by controlling the minds and money's of the people. The heads of the Illuminati are a number of the riches families around the world. They control most of the banks, politics, Roman Catholic Churches, Christine Churches and corporations around the Globe. And are presently trying to gain world wide control of the Earth and all upon the Earth. One of its methods of control is to pollute man's body weakening his physical essence then pollute and control man's mental thoughts (T.V., Radio, False Religion, Newspapers, ect…) which will prevent man from knowing of her/his spiritual essence therefore rendering them as a spiritless beings, whom can only act out the will of others (like a robot) and not his/her own free will. The taking away of a man/woman's spiritual essence is to take away their strongest means of bringing change to their life by way of their connection with the Almighty Creator.

Conclusion

After achieving a healthier life style you will have given yourself more peace of mind, can deal with work and home problems much better than before and can excel in home and work activities much better than before. Others will be attractted to you and like to be as you are. Also you will have better relations with your mate and a higher spiritual awareness.

If you agree with the information contained in this book then memorize and learn it, then use it in your every day life and you shall see a change in your life for the better! You should also do your own research into the various area's of concern so that you can obtain more proof of the facts brought forth in these writings.

The Creator's truth is to be freely shared by all. So what ever truth you learn always pass it to another so that he/she can raise their conscious state of being and move toward a higher knowledge of Self and the Creator.

A good slave is one that is unhealthy and has a low conscious state of mind and they will always be controlled and can never live their life to the fullest until they are healthy and have raises their conscious state of mind.

You have your entire life to perfect your self Physically, Mentally and Spiritually. This is a lot of time so use it wisely and don't waste it or just let it pass you by. You can improve your way of life a great deal by making an effort to learn and follow the things that you have chose to be truths in your life. Send out Meditative Prayer to the Creator for the creation of a more righteous world. And pray for me that I may receive the energy to continue bringing forth righteous knowledge to the people.

When I talk to people on this subject matter, I've spoke on things that I did not know of, seconds before, when I began to speak. This is one proof to me that the knowledge of all things is contained within the mind (mental, intellect). And all we need to do is to search for it. The Creator instilled this knowledge in each human being, so "Know Thyself " and you shall know all. The mind connected to spirit brings forth knowledge of all things. All humans have a mind spirit connection but we don't use it.

Under the same law that states matter can not be created or destroyed. There is no such thing as new knowledge, there is only the lack of knowledge (or lack of understanding). "Know Thyself ".

You now have the Knowledge of your Ancestors what will you do with it!!!

Dedication

I dedicate this book to my mother "Minnie G. Forrest" and all of humanity, whom are searching for and wish to know the TRUTH's in life.

Please pass this knowledge to all of mankind, for it will create a "New and Better World".

Work Sheets

Instructions:
Please use the following pages to note down all the new truths that you have come to acknowledge to yourself as true. And work each day to continue listing all the new truths you have learned, and practice them in your life everyday. Once your table of truths is established, you will have a code of ethics for the way you should live your life, that can be past on to your children, family and friends and the world.

Physical Truths

Mental Truths

Spiritual Truths

REFERENCES:

BOOK TITTLE	AUTHOR
Stolen Legacy	George G.M. James
From The Browder Files	Anthony T Browder
Historical Origin of Christianity	Walter Williams
Signs & Symbols of Primordial Man	Albert Churchward
THE ANKH	NU ANKH AMEN
Ageless Wisdom Guide to Healing	Ra Un Nefer Amen
Initiation into Egyptian Yoga	Dr. Muata Abhaya Ashby
The Science of Melanin	T. OWENS MOORE PH.D.
Light from Ancient Africa	Na'im Akbar Ph.D.
The Finding of the Third Eye	Vera Stanley Alder
Initiation Into Egyptian Yoga	Dr. Muata Abhaya Ashby
The Mystical Teachings of The Ausarian Resurrection	Dr. Muata Abhaya Ashby
Africa is not a country it is a continent	Dr. Autor Lewin
Your Days are numbered (numerology)	Floerence Campbell
The Cycle of Time	Dr. Muata Abhaya Ashby
From Egypt to Greece	Dr. Muata Abhaya Ashby
The Hidden Properties of Matter	Dr. Muata Abhaya Ashby
Egyptian Proverbs	Dr. Muata Abhaya Ashby
African Holistic Health	Llaila O. Afrika (Doctor)
Egyptian Yoga Volume II	Dr. Muata Abhaya Ashby
The Book Your Church Doesn't Want You to Read	Tim C. Leedom
The Kybalion Hermetic Philosophy	Three Initiates
Heal Thyself (for health and longevity)	By Queen Afua
AS A MAN THINKETH	James Allen
Songs of The Stars (The lore of a Zulu Shaman)	Vusamazulu Credo Mutwa
Pyramid Energy(philosophy of God science of man)	Hardy & Killick
Cosmic Science of The Ancient Masters	Professor Hilton Hotema
Pre-Existence of Man	Professor Hilton Hotema
The Mysterious SPHINX	Professor Hilton Hotema
The Magic World	Professor Hilton Hotema
Creation Cosmic Radiation	Professor Hilton Hotema
Melanin The Chemical Key to Black's Greatness	Carol Barns (Sr. Research chemist)
The Sorcerer's Crossing	By Taisha Abelar
Predictions for the Year 2000 & Beyond	By Gus Vandermeer
The Only Astrology Book You'll Ever Need	Joanna Martine Woolfolk
Sedona Starseed	Raymond Mardyks

Science of Being	Eugene Fersen
Killing In The Name Of Love	Alvin Morrow
The Pleiadian Agenda	Barbara Hand Clow
The Science of Psychic Healing	"Yogi" Ramacharaka

References Continued:

Lectures & Conversations

Dr Albert Blair
Dr. Africa
Dr. Finch
Miss Dr. Doni Ani
Steve Cokely
Tony Martin
Dr. Ben
Dr. King
Dr. Jack Feider
Rev. Phalintine
Henry DeBernardo
Ashra Kwesi
Dr. Whitaker
Dr. D.M. Berry "Master Teacher "
Osiris Stargod
Serud
Kalif Amen-Ra
Nu Ankh NTR Amen
Bro. Dawud
Tony Martin
Doc-B
Steve Cokely
C. Mulling
Gregg Braden

POEMS

Sunshine Moonlight

Sunshine, Moonlight please stay
Bring light, to my life, each day
Your light, has shown me the way

Your rays are like strands of gold
So precious, everlasting and bold

I can hear your light rays as they travel through the air
Like musical chimes, oh what a pair

I smell your light rays as I pass a flower
You are nature, oh what power

I wonder how did you get up in the sky so far
But one thing I know, you are two beautiful stars

Your energies, they fill my heart
Giving strength, to make a new start

Your vibrations, I feel in my soul
This feeling, will never, grow old

With out you, I'd be so cold
My life, would end you know

So always be there for me
Sending your loving rays to me

Your light is so bright
It propels my soul into flight

And the closer I get to you
The more I remember all that you do

You bring life to this world
As your energy rains down in swirls

And if you ever go away
I thank you for the life you have brought us each day

So on that day that the Creator calls you home
I will be so all alone

No Sunlight to lift me up each day
No Moonlight to illuminate my dreams as I lay

So beautiful Sun and Moon always be their for me

By: Kevin Forrest

Super Energy in Me

The Creator has bestowed in me
An energy, that makes me be
A superman, oh can't you see

My Melanin is the processor, can't you see
That pulls down this super energy
And stimulates my spirituality
Now I am free

This energy lives on eternally in me
It will show me things through my Third-Eye
From the future and past, can't you see

I can feel this energy rising up threw me
Taking me to places, I could never be, without this energy

When this energy reaches my mind
I evolve into one of the super kind

Now its time
To remove the blinds
And heal the world, one more time

By: Kevin Forrest

Why So Much Pain

I don't know why the world is so cold
I think it's got me in a choke hold

It's got me sitting in the sunshine
Trying to ease the pain that I feel inside

I step back and try to breath
It's got me begging oh lord please

Now I'm sitting in the sunshine
Trying to pull down energies to ease my mind

Then a ray of light showed me a plan
How I could be a better man

I healed my mind
And it feels is so fine

Now I see the world in a different light
And once again I can sleep at night

Come world and follow me
So we can spread this love, over mountains and out to sea

This love will flow threw galaxies
If you try it, you will see

Once again the world is so nice
This love is so thick you can cut it with a knife

No babies crying in the night
No smog blocking out the light

No chemicals causing pain
And our bodies can rest again

No jealousy between sister and brother
Now we can love one another

By: Kevin Forrest

Fake Knowledge

You know I went to college
And they gave me fake knowledge

They didn't stimulate my mine
They just wasted all my time

Why did I waste away those years
Now all I have to show is tears
Oh I feel so low
From my head down to my toes

And know I am blind
All I see is this rhyme

Know I am trying to heal my mind
And take away the blinds
Sending energies threw my spine
In an attempt to heal my mind

That's why I am standing in the Sun
Trying to load my gun
I'm gonna blast away the fear
Yes you know this my dear

Oh please send to me
Some real knowledge "G"

So I can be
The man I'm suppose to be

Stimulate my third-eye
And take me to the spiritual sky's

By: Kevin Forrest

THE
AFRICAN
HOLISTIC
MOTIVATIONAL
HEALING
GUIDE

"Heal Our African Nation"

Book Order Form

To order your copy please send this order form to:

Kevin M. Forrest
761 North 80th Street
E. St. Louis, IL. 62203

Please send:
_______ Copies of "The African Holistic Motivational Healing Guide"
(Heal Our African Nation)

Send Money Order or Cashiers Check for $ 9.95 plus $ 3.00 shipping & handling to: Kevin Forrest, 761 North 80th Street, E. St. Louis, IL. 62203 Add one dollar for each additional book ordered.

Name:____

Address:____

City:___________________________State:________Zip:________

THE
AFRICAN
HOLISTIC
MOTIVATIONAL
HEALING
GUIDE

"Heal Our African Nation"

Book Order Form

To order your copy please send this order form to:

Kevin M. Forrest
761 North 80th Street
E. St. Louis, IL. 62203

Please send:

_______ Copies of "The African Holistic Motivational Healing Guide"
(Heal Our African Nation)

Send Money Order or Cashiers Check for $ 9.95 plus $ 3.00 shipping & handling to: Kevin Forrest, 761 North 80th Street, E. St. Louis, IL. 62203 Add one dollar for each additional book ordered.

Name:____

Address:____

City:___________________________State:_______Zip:________
